NURSING
WISELY

NURSING WISELY: How to Build a Nursing Career That Is Worthwhile, Interesting, Sustainable, Empowered, and Limitless by Putting Yourself First

Copyright © 2023 by Mary Ghazarian

This is a work of creative nonfiction. Some parts have been fictionalized in varying degrees, for various purposes. The events and conversations in this book have been set down to the best of the author's ability, although some names and details have been changed to protect the privacy of individuals.

All rights reserved. No part of this book may be reproduced or used in any manner without written permission of the copyright owner except for the use of quotations in a book review.

The author and publisher of this book have used their best efforts in preparing this material. While every attempt has been made to verify the information provided in this book, neither the author nor the publisher assumes any responsibility for errors, omissions, inaccuracies, or results attained upon applying the contents of the book

The author and publisher or any other contributor to this book shall in no event be liable for any loss, or other damages, including, but not limited to special, incidental, consequential or other damages. As always, the direct and specific advice of a competent professional that specializes in the reader's specific circumstances should be sought.

For information about special discounts for bulk purchases or other inquiries contact: info@maryghazarian.com

Cover and Interior design by Olivier Darbonville
Edited by Lisa MacDonald

ISBN 978-1-7390513-2-7 (hardcover)
ISBN 978-1-7390513-1-0 (softcover)
ISBN 978-1-7390513-0-3 (ebook)

NURSING
WISELY

HOW TO BUILD A **NURSING CAREER**
THAT IS WORTHWHILE, INTERESTING,
SUSTAINABLE, EMPOWERED, AND
LIMITLESS **BY PUTTING YOURSELF FIRST**

MARY GHAZARIAN MN, NP-PHC

DEDICATION

For my *husband* for keeping my eyes open to possibilities,
and providing the support to pursue them.
For my *mother* for listening and leading by example.
For my *mentors* for seeing potential in me that I didn't know was there.

CONTENTS

FOREWORD 11

INTRODUCTION 13

MY NURSING STORY 25

MODULE 1. Creating a Worthwhile Career — 41
1. What Makes Nursing Worthwhile? — 42
2. Define Your Values — 49
3. Identify Your Niche — 53
4. Reverse Engineering Your Nursing Career — 60
5. Set Worthwhile Goals — 65
6. Achieve Your Goals — 75

MODULE 2. Keeping Your Career Interesting — 81
7. Risks of a Boring Career — 82
8. Creating Interest — 86
9. Opportunity Knocks — 93
10. Lateral Moves — 98
11. How *Not* to Keep Things Interesting — 104

MODULE 3. Sustaining a Successful Career — 109
12. What is Sustainability? — 110
13. Time Freedom — 112
14. Creating Connections: Support, Fellowship, and Networking — 119
15. Financial Sustainability — 125
16. Legacy — 130

MODULE 4. Empowered: Embracing Lifelong Learning — 135
- 17 Nursing Empowerment — 136
- 18 Knowledge — 137
- 19 Creativity — 141
- 20 Advocacy — 144
- 21 Experience and Resilience — 151
- 22 Embrace Feedback — 156

MODULE 5. Building a Career Without Limits! — 161
- 23 Limiting Beliefs in Nursing — 162
- 24 Nursing Income Beliefs — 166
- 25 Nursing Status Beliefs — 175
- 26 The Business of Nursing — 178
- 27 Imposter Syndrome and Fear of Failure — 181

MODULE 6. You: Living Authentically and Self-Care! — 187
- 27 Your Authentic Opportunity — 188
- 28 Your Professional Image — 191
- 29 Your Time — 197
- 30 Your Mental and Spiritual Health — 202
- 31 Your Physical Health — 215
- 32 Your Personal Identity — 224

Nursing WISELY: Stories from Successful Nurses — 227
- Claudia Mariano, Former Nurse Practitioner — 227
- Dr. Sonja Mitrevska Schwartzbach, CRNA — 229
- Melane Mullings — 232
- Stacey Roles, RN MScN PhD Psychotherapist — 235

EPILOGUE   241

BONUS: ORGANIZATIONAL RECRUITMENT AND RETENTION WITH NURSING WISELY   243

SELECTED BIBLIOGRAPHY / WORKS CITED   245

ABOUT THE AUTHOR   249

FOREWORD

"Learning is a process where knowledge is presented to us, then shaped through understanding, discussion and reflection."

—Paulo Friere

I MET MARY THROUGH AN ONLINE nursing independent practice interest group which she was hosting. I witnessed Mary leading and coaching a thousand of her peers on how to grow a nursing-based business of their own. Her passion for breaking boundaries and expanding possibilities was palpable and inspiring. Next, I was introduced to Mary's *Nursing WISELY* career framework that recognizes and focuses on the unique needs of the individual nurse across their career trajectory.

Nurses are so engulfed in our work to improve the lives of others, that we seldom devote time for self-reflection. We undervalue and fail to prioritize the time it takes to learn from the lessons we are experiencing. As a result, we miss valuable opportunities—that could propel us forward in both our personal and professional lives—for self-care and professional caring.

Nursing WISELY outlines the key components to achieving a successful nursing career.

Mary effectively does this through the sharing of relatable stories, hard won lessons, and hands-on exercises. Approach *Nursing* WISELY with an open mind and willing heart. Take the time to do the reflective exercises at the end of each chapter, to support and reveal your authentic and transformational journey towards the lessons that can emerge for you.

Nursing WISELY's foundation resonates with me.

- You cannot meet the needs of others, if you do not meet your own needs first.
- You can overcome limitations.
- You are worth it.
- You can achieve your dreams.

It is empowering to understand that today's challenges and limitations are tomorrow's opportunities. You can create positive change in the world throughout your nursing career by harnessing and leveraging *your* unique blend of talents, abilities, experiences, and points of view.

Embrace opportunity, growth and learning. Secure a mentor for coaching. Get actively involved in professional organizations. Have courageous conversations. Challenge the status quo. Be a disruptive innovator.

Reading *Nursing WISELY* is the first step to expanding the horizon of your nursing career, creating limitless potential to make a positive impact on your patients, the nursing community, and society at large.

Invest in yourself through self-reflection, awareness, and discovery. Catapult your joy, influence and impact. Strengthen or resuscitate your personal and professional passion to leverage your expertise, compassion and future legacies.

I wish you great success.

Dr. Michelle Acorn,

[signature]

DNP, NP PHC/Adult, MN/ACNP, BScN/PHCNP, FCAN, FAAN, FFNMRCSI, CGNC
Past President Nurse Practitioner Association of Ontario
Former Ontario Provincial Chief Nursing Officer
Current Inaugural Chief Nurse of the International Council of Nurses

INTRODUCTION

Do you remember the feeling you had when you were first accepted to nursing school? Pride? Possibility? Panic?

For me, there was a feeling of certainty. The future was no longer unknown. I had a path and a destination.

"*Congratulations...*" I pumped the letter high into the air! As a high school student, there was no greater accomplishment I could imagine. My future was set.

The following weekend I drove from my mother's house in Ontario to my father's home in Quebec to share the news in person. I beamed as I announced that I would be attending "Harvard of the North," Queen's University in Kingston, Ontario. My father had supported my brother to attend Bible college a few years prior, so without a second thought, I asked for help with tuition.

"Women don't need to go to university, that's what husbands are for," was his reply.

Immigrant parents are typically thought of as pushing their children to become doctors, lawyers, or a member of another valued profession. I didn't imagine that my own immigrant father held archaic gender values.

My nursing career could have died there. Taking a year off after high school for some dedicated husband hunting might have sounded fun to any other 17-year-old. But, having witnessed the lack of financial security my mother faced after the divorce, I vowed to make my own way without my father's support. I was going to build a successful nursing career at all costs.

With no savings to speak of, I survived nursing school with the help of bursaries, student loans, and part-time work at a women's shelter. After a grueling four years and a final placement in remote Moose Factory, Ontario, traditional territory of the Moose Cree First Nation, I snagged my first nursing position in a prestigious downtown hospital and set off for the big city.

Fast forward to the reality of daily nurse life. Echoes of the cloud nine moment I felt when I first opened my nursing school acceptance letter were everywhere – in the flash of blood in a perfectly placed butterfly needle, bringing someone back to life after a successful resuscitation, and the general satisfaction at the end of a shift of knowing my patients and I survived 12 more hours. Sweet dopamine.

Those successes led to a sort of pathologic altruism. In my attempt to be the "best nurse" and the "best colleague," I gave more of myself than I could afford. I skipped breaks, didn't take vacation, held my bladder for 12+ hours multiple times a week, volunteered for every opportunity, said yes to every request, and stayed behind to help with emergencies at shift change. Repeatedly, over a five-year period, I burnt myself out for an annual raise of 15 cents an hour.

Thankfully, that's not how my nursing career story ended and it's not how I want *your* story to end either.

You may have picked up this book because you're bored or fed up or looking for a change, something to propel you forward. Maybe *Nursing WISELY* was recommended by someone who wants to see you realize your potential. Or perhaps you were just curious. Either way, this book was meant for you.

Nurses have an identity that forms almost immediately as they enter school. First peers call you "Nurse," and then you have unique experiences you can't easily talk about at the dinner table. You start to hide parts of yourself in your home and social life. The only ones you feel can relate are your nursing peers.

When another nurse demands help, we make room for the chaos.

We hold space for one another over a beverage or a breakroom pizza. We provide advice we wish we could follow, but don't. We bond. We create strong relationships that dictate whether we will take an extra shift depending on who is working. Nursing is difficult, but most nurses appear to have it together. Meanwhile, most feel like an imposter and look at each other wondering how they're holding it together. What's the secret to their success? What do they know that I don't?

In *Nursing WISELY*, I share the story of how I created my ideal career when I followed my own advice, reclaimed my personal identity, and prioritized myself. My hope is that reading my experience will help you to also create your success story. We have the power to redefine nursing and help the next generation of nurses that follow. We can save them from the systemic issues that have plagued nurses around the world for generations. Patient-centered care will not be sacrificed but better enabled by putting ourselves first.

I want you to explore: the feeling of being able to leave work at work, of working in a unit that is never understaffed, of gaining energy from healthy nutrition and bio-breaks, and of being awarded with money rather than a service pin.

If you have an entrepreneurial spirit, I want you to know the feeling of personally signing the pay cheques for the employees of a nursing-based business you own. I want you to experience the feelings associated with achieving your dreams, feelings you may not have experienced in your career to this point, but that are achievable.

While I do share my story and the stories of other successful nurses throughout this book, *Nursing WISELY* isn't intended to be a collection of nursing stories, a textbook detailing how to insert the most painless IV (although I am excellent with a hard stick), or a journey through the daily experiences of shift work. Instead, you will find stories and prompts that guide you to tap into your own wisdom for a great nursing career.

Nurses come from diverse backgrounds but we are all striving for something. Only you know what that "something" is but this book will help you to achieve your ideal nursing career if you are willing to do the work it takes to get there. As a nursing career coach, I teach nurses, like you, how to build a nursing career that is **w**orthwhile, **i**nteresting, **s**ustainable, **e**mpowered, and **l**imitless by putting themselves first. If you're interested in learning how to build this type of nursing career, then you are in the right place!

You'll soon be on your way to discovering the secrets of a successful career in nursing, beyond what they teach you in nursing school! Together we'll build your best practice guideline to your professional nursing career.

How to Read this Book

This is not a nursing textbook, full of abstract concepts that you'll struggle to read through. You'll find only the advice I wish I'd had before starting my nursing career.

To get the most out of this book, I recommend:

1. Read actively. Write notes in the margins, underline or highlight key points. You won't want to re-sell this book, so go ahead and mark it up! (Keep a journal close by if you're an e-book fan)
2. Mark or record pages you'd like to return to.
3. In each module you'll have the opportunity to complete exercises that will help you move forward in your nursing career. Answer writing prompts in this book in whatever format works for you.
4. Write by hand instead of keeping electronic notes. Hand writing your thoughts increases retention and allows the subconscious to work through goals, problems, and thoughts at night while you sleep! You'll be surprised how answers surface as you continue to move toward your goals a year from now.
5. Don't limit yourself to writing bullet points. Get creative. Draw diagrams and pictures. Allow your ideas to flow.

INTRODUCTION   **17**

6. Answer questions honestly. You don't have to show them to anyone.
7. Get stuck on a question? Ask yourself: What if you *did* know? What would your answer be then?
8. Can't answer the questions on your own? Consider hiring a career coach to help you get past a mental block.
9. Check in with yourself periodically. Ask yourself – "How am I doing? What has surprised me? What can I implement/change today to move closer to my goals?"
10. Read the modules in whatever order most interests or serves you. Everyone's journey is unique.

What is *Nursing WISELY?*

You decided to become a nurse!

You registered for your program, paid the fees, and gave up most of your spare time for two to four years - or longer! Maybe you even repeated the process for a Master's or PhD. You learned the health lingo, the history, the theories, the science, the art, and the norms. You stayed up late with a bottle of wine or pot of coffee to write and edit papers only your professors or TAs read. You completed clinical hours while your friends partied and slept in and, you passed grueling exam after grueling exam.

You may have had to overcome additional challenges, including a learning disability, mental health condition, or long-term chronic illness. You may also have been raising a family, caring for aging parents, or navigating tumultuous relationships. Were you working with a tight budget, working multiple jobs while studying full-time? Perhaps you found yourself accessing food banks and other social supports? Post-secondary education is also a time for discovering or learning to express your gender or sexual identity while in a program, institution, or city that may not have accepted you for who you were. And yet, you persevered!

With your school pass on the books, you registered for an official licensing exam to prove you completed your fully accredited program with a sound understanding of nursing.

Finally - you passed *for real!*

Despite the tears, the sleepless nights, and the world that seemed to conspire against you - you made it! Your regulatory body determined it wasn't just a fluke that you graduated in the first place, and awarded you with the title of "Nurse."

> Deep sigh of relief!
> Pop the champagne!
> Clink! Clink!
> You made it!

If you're still a student or considering nursing as a career - envision yourself in celebration!

No one except your nursing peers can quite understand the ups and downs of becoming a nurse. You joined the ranks of an exclusive club of life-saving professionals and, you didn't just take on a title - you took on *a new identity*. Despite all of your time as a student, you may not have been prepared for what came next.

- Did you accept the first available job because it provided a stable pay cheque and pension? Are you still there?
- Did you spend the beginning of your career at the bedside in the hospital to nail down your skills or go directly into that other area of practice you loved like public health? Or did you continue directly into your master's degree or other higher education?
- If you started nursing in a hospital, long-term care facility or institution, do you stay there to maintain your nursing skills instead of a less traditional role away from the bedside, and into management or being an entrepreneur?

More than once, you may have asked yourself: "Is this really what I'm passionate about?" "Do I want to spend the majority of my waking hours doing this?" "Does my job bring me meaning?" "How do I discover the right nursing job for me?"

It's a big world out there! Your dream nursing job may not even exist yet! It certainly can't exist unless you know what qualities your dream job has and open your mind up to the possibilities.

Being a successful full-time nurse is really hard. It takes diligence and resilience, day in and day out. You are the owner of your nursing license, the self-marketer, the cheerleader, the naysayer, the accountant, the billpayer, the dog/cat/human/other parent, and overseer of all of the things that have to be done. Oh, and you also need to enjoy your life along the way!

Despite my focus on success, I got everything *wrong* for the first ten years of my professional nursing career. Whatever the opposite of *Nursing WISELY* was, I was doing that!

Freedom and fulfillment in your nursing career are possible. I'm going to tell you how I found it and how you can too!

In this book, I share the advice I wish I had to guide me, but wasn't included in my undergraduate or graduate nursing education. It is advice I have given one-on-one to nursing colleagues over coffee and to nursing career coaching clients, and now I pass on to you!

There are endless reasons (or excuses) why we don't learn these things in school. Professors and colleagues have told me:

1. The most important things nurses need to know are basic nursing skills.
2. Nurses mainly work for hospitals.
3. Nurses are employees and don't run their own businesses.
4. There is too much to teach and too little time to spend more than a few hours on career planning.
5. Nurses learn best when they are thrown into the fire.

These are all myths. This book will prove to you that there is more to your career than being thrown to the wolves and "surviving" the nursing culture of eating their young.

The truth is, little is included about career alternatives in the nursing curriculum; few nurse educators have MBAs or experience outside of traditional nursing roles and the largest source of public funding for nursing education exists to generate staff for hospitals and long-term care settings.

Healthcare systems that do not demonstrate the value of nurses are unsustainable. Hospitals need an endless supply of nurses because of high turnover—turnover that may be avoidable with adequate staffing and remuneration.

So, what's a nurse to do? Put yourself first! It's not enough to advocate for your patients. You need to know how to advocate for yourself, your nursing colleagues, your collective rights, and your compensation!

It's time to discover the opportunities in nursing that are right for you. Opportunities in nursing are ever-expanding. Multi-passionate nurses have established successful careers in the areas of nursing informatics, nurse health coaching, nurse-led clinics, nurse health system navigation, cosmetic nursing, nursing homes, healthcare product development and nursing wealth coaches.

It is possible to combine specialties and interests to create new nursing career opportunities that are personally fulfilling *and* contribute to society in ways that are essential to individuals, families, communities, and corporations.

Pursue career opportunities that align with your values, goals, and interests. Create your ideal career, birthed from your authentic interests, and then grow it.

- Are you unsure what your next career step should be?
- Are self-limiting beliefs getting in the way of being able to realize your dreams, goals, or personal vision?

- Are you stuck in a stage of your career that is no longer fulfilling, and need help moving forward?
- Are you seeking work-life balance? Or, do you need help deciding which new responsibilities to take on and which old ones to shed?
- Are you considering how to reduce your workload to make it more manageable?
- Are you preparing for retirement or another significant life change?
- Are you considering ditching nursing altogether?

Whether you are a novice, mid-career, or expert nurse, to create your career path, you need to be aware of what you enjoy, what is available, and where you want to be in 3, 5, 10, and 20 years from now. Does that seem too distant? Research shows we make better long-term decisions when we visually see an older version of ourselves.[1]

STOP AND THINK

Use an app to age yourself. Print a copy, and let "future you" talk about their life experience. Imagine all the things you had to do to get there and imagine the satisfaction of a having a nursing career on your own terms.

As you work through the *Nursing WISELY* modules, you will:
- gain clarity
- build a nursing career path you didn't realize was possible
- feel more confident about your nursing career and status as a nurse

---

1 Hershfield et al. (2011). Increasing Saving Behavior Through Age-Progressed Renderings of the Future Self. *Journal of Marketing Research*, 48(SPL), S23–S37. https://doi.org/10.1509/jmkr.48.SPL.S23

- find the light at the end of the nursing burn-out tunnel
- create a support network who will keep you accountable to your goals
- decrease anxiety about your career
- evoke a vision and plan for taking action
- and, learn the essentials not taught in nursing school!

You'll have the opportunity to identify what fills you with anxiety and explore what energizes you!

Implementing change and taking the time to reflect on what you truly want is hard! If it wasn't, you would've done it by now! But I promise you, it's easier than having to secretly grab a bite of a protein bar while sitting on the toilet - having finally escaped to the only available private washroom. Yes, I have done it, but you don't have to!

What uncertainties are holding you back? Do you think pursuing more education is too time-consuming and expensive? Are you worried that advancing your career will take time away from friends and family? Maybe you don't love academics and have had your fill of nursing knowledge? Whatever you are feeling or thinking, *Nursing WISELY* can help you to throw self-limiting beliefs out the window so you can pursue and achieve your dreams!

Learn to Nurse WISELY
The acronym stands for:

Worthwhile	My career pursuits are worthwhile.
Interesting	My career pursuits interest me and keep my attention.
Sustainable	My career is something I can see myself pursuing into retirement.
Empowered	My career is empowered and involves lifelong learning.
Limitless	My career goals have no boundaries or limiting beliefs.
You	My career comes from a place of authenticity and meets my needs first.

EXERCISE: Rate yourself

Rate yourself in the six areas of nursing career success. How do you feel about your nursing career *right now* on a scale of 1 to 10. (1 = not at all and 10 = absolutely)

Periodically return to this exercise to assess areas of strength and opportunity in your career.

Remember, a *career* is a long-term endeavor, something you build towards and work upon every day, while a *job* is something you do for money.

My career is worthwhile.

1 — 2 — 3 — 4 — 5 — 6 — 7 — 8 — 9 — 10

My career pursuits interest me and keep my attention.

1 — 2 — 3 — 4 — 5 — 6 — 7 — 8 — 9 — 10

My career is something I can see myself pursuing into retirement and beyond.

1 — 2 — 3 — 4 — 5 — 6 — 7 — 8 — 9 — 10

My career is empowered and involves lifelong learning.

1 — 2 — 3 — 4 — 5 — 6 — 7 — 8 — 9 — 10

My career goals have no boundaries and are not held back by limiting beliefs.

1 — 2 — 3 — 4 — 5 — 6 — 7 — 8 — 9 — 10

My career comes from a place of authenticity and meets my needs first.

1 — 2 — 3 — 4 — 5 — 6 — 7 — 8 — 9 — 10

For anything you rated less than 10, what is one thing you can do to increase the score?

Not sure? Working through the exercises in this book will bring you closer to a 10.

MY NURSING STORY

WITH FRIENDLY EYES BEHIND THICK-RIMMED glasses and an air of genuine curiosity, the impressively titled Nursing Innovation Project Manager asked, "Why did you get into nursing?"

I was three years into my nursing career and found myself sitting in a boardroom filled with ten of the most brilliant bedside nurses I had ever met. As the recipients of a prestigious nursing fellowship, we were gathered together for a unique opportunity. For three months, we would be paid to work an "80-20" split. Eighty percent of our working hours would be dedicated to our usual positions, mine was with the hospital's Nursing Resource Team (NRT), and twenty percent to the projects we had described in our fellowship applications. We would also meet every two weeks for mentorship.

We took turns answering our mentor's question. The other nurses had impressive and selfless origin stories. Most had grown up knowing they would become nurses. They had family members they admired who were nurses or they had an experience as a patient that led them to becoming a nurse. They loved to help people. They wanted to make a difference in the lives of patients. They wanted to dedicate their lives to service.

One nurse described her experience of organizing mission trips to her home country. She delivered medical supplies and set up clinics in remote areas to bring healthcare to those in need. The story was so compelling that she was featured in a promotional video for the hospital a few months later!

Then, there was my answer to why I became a nurse. "To make money," I said.

17-year-old me decided to get into nursing for the big bucks! Cue the video of me with dollar signs in my eyes diving into a pool of gold doubloons! Ok, I didn't get into nursing to become a millionaire but I *was* in search of financial security. While it may have been easier to lie, I put my truth out there in front of a room full of people I barely knew.

If a want for financial security is your truth too, let it be known! You deserve to earn a sustainable living and have more financial security than living pay cheque to pay cheque.

Money continues to be a strong driver in my career, but with a firm understanding of the financial aspects of this career, space has opened for other motivations, passions, and values. Along the way, I developed values like work-life balance and mental health. I also value achieving financial security in a way that is satisfying and does not lead to an unhealthy relationship with work, food, alcohol, or other vices. And, I have a passion for helping other nurses to build healthy lives and careers too.

We all need money. Unfortunately, I was pursuing "shiny opportunities" in hopes of more money and security from jobs or organizations that could provide neither. A valuable lesson I have learned is that having a deeper motivation for nursing will sustain your career over the long term.

Before nursing

With its large birch trees, fragrant lavender bushes, a bountiful vegetable garden, swimming pool, basketball hoop in the driveway, and a hill that was great for tobogganing, my childhood home left nothing to be desired. My idyllic childhood came to an end when my family of six was torn apart by divorce. My father and two brothers stayed in my childhood home. I moved a province away into the basement of a family member's house with my mother and sister.

Having been promised by my father that she would never need a dime of her own money, my mother had given up nursing school in her early twenties and taken on a career as a stay-at-home mom. After the divorce, in need of a way to support us, my mother went to night school to become a Personal Support Worker. A year later, with certification in hand, my mother remarried and we moved again. The new house featured a dirt-floored basement and crumbling plaster walls - a far cry from the quality red brick construction of my childhood home built by the hands of my grandfather.

Shortly after the move, my stepfather was injured in a motorcycle accident. Given my mother's salary was only slightly better than minimum wage, I witnessed the struggle as she supported us on her meager income. I could only imagine the crushing weight of being the sole earner through this life transition. She left early in the morning, returned late at night, and often stayed up cooking meals, making lunches, and doing chores. I imagine she collapsed into her bed for just a few hours before getting up to do it again the next day.

Before my parent's divorce, I had lofty dreams of becoming an actress. As an eight-year-old, I daydreamed of walking through the mall and being spotted by a talent agent who would whisk me away to Hollywood for a leading role. After the divorce, I decided I just wanted to survive. My goal was to be able to be self-sufficient no matter what came my way. I vowed never to have to depend on a partner to financially support me.

In high school, my teachers hammered home the message that going to university was the ticket to financial independence. I didn't know what that meant exactly, because no one in my family had ever gone to university. But I took their advice and took the university stream of courses, sneaking in a drama course for fun.

As application deadlines approached, I was overwhelmed. I didn't understand my options. What was the difference between college and university? One was two years and the other was four. One cost less and the other more but, I didn't understand *why*.

I visited the guidance counselor for advice. "What do *you* want to do?" she asked. I didn't have an answer. All I knew was that financial security was important to me. I wanted to pursue a job that was secure with earning potential and I wanted someone to tell me how to get that but, was too embarrassed to ask. Instead, I clammed up and left the office.

I searched for answers in university brochures and on the internet where I wouldn't be judged for asking "stupid" questions. I entered search terms like, "What careers are in demand?" and "What careers make the most money?" I reviewed my options.

Bachelor of Arts.	What profession would I join with that degree?
Engineering.	Never heard of it and took drama instead of physics, so no.
Business.	Too vague.
Science.	Too broad.
Nursing.	Nurse was a familiar word.

Both my mother and grandmother had gone to nursing school but both left to get married. Nursing had a clear path in terms of both profession and earning money and, the internet told me nurses were in demand, so I felt there would be job security.

I spent hours trying to understand the difference between a college education leading to a Registered Practical Nurse (RPN) certification versus a university education leading to a Registered Nurse (RN) certification. Both certifications sounded the same to me. A nurse was a nurse, was a nurse as far as I knew. Even worse, I didn't know what a nurse actually *did*.

A shorter period in school with less financial investment to become a nurse sounded like a no-brainer but, I knew there must be a catch. With earning potential being my primary driver, I searched for the average earnings of an RPN versus an RN. I discovered both earned more money than I could truly understand based on my history of minimum wage part-time work, but in the end, it was clear that RNs earned more than RPNs.

Application deadlines arrived. The hundreds of dollars required for application fees was a huge amount of money for me. I submitted applications to Bachelor of Nursing programs at University of Toronto, Queen's University, and McGill University.

My application to the University of Toronto returned with a disappointing, "We regret to inform you..." but I was accepted to the other two schools. My investment paid off. I chose Queen's University in Kingston, Ontario so I could live with my aunt and uncle and save on rent.

My next challenge was to figure out how to pay for university. I had unimpressive savings, no college fund, and my mother certainly couldn't afford it, so I approached my father. He nearly disowned me for asking for help. Thank goodness for student loans.

Undergrad

"Look to your left. Look to your right. By the end of the semester one of these people will no longer be here," said my esteemed professor/fortune-teller on the first day of my undergraduate nursing experience. After a brief glance in each direction, my classmates and I sank low in our chairs but as the professor predicted, each class had more empty seats than the last. Our starting class of 200 dwindled down to a class half the size over the course of four years.

My goal to become self-sufficient fueled my determination. No matter how much I longed to sleep in, rather than attend clinical placement that started before sunrise, I attended classes faithfully. (These were the days before recorded lectures.) I never broke the dress code for clinical placements (no jeans in the hospital and steel blue scrubs only), and took advantage of all learning opportunities. Not even the embarrassment of fainting the first time I witnessed an emergency chest tube insertion stopped me from showing up.

At the advice of my professors, I applied for jobs in my final semester and had a job before I graduated. I completed my degree thousands of dollars in debt, but met my goal of self-sufficiency by the age of 21.

Early career

My first nursing position was with the Nursing Resource Team at a metropolitan teaching hospital that had two locations. NRT was the respectable term for "float pool." Prior to every shift, before choosing which subway line to get on, I would call a messaging system that would tell me which hospital and unit I was going to. Sometimes, by the time I reached the unit, I would be redirected to another unit or the other hospital. Learning to roll with life's punches during my parents' divorce helped me thrive in the NRT.

During my first few years of work, I looked for an area of nursing that would make me feel fulfilled, but never pursued opportunities I knew would make me happy. I was afraid of disappointment, failure, and felt unworthy of actual happiness in my career. I yearned to specialize in psychiatry or eating disorders, but held back from asking my manager to work on those units.

"What if they think I'm ungrateful for all the training they gave me in the other units? What if they fire me?" I thought.

There was a lot of emotional baggage driving my career in those early days. I was fearful of rejection, had feelings of unworthiness, and suffered from imposter syndrome. I didn't want anyone to take away my hard-earned financial security and became so focused on gaining experience and being a good employee that I didn't even take time off for vacation.

Within two years, I climbed my imagined bedside nursing ladder - moving from floor nursing to the ER and then to the Intensive Care Unit. At each more specialized level, I noticed a difference in the way physician colleagues treated me. I decided they were on the imaginary ladder with me too. Physicians gave me more respect as my expertise became more specialized. Those little ego boosts kept me going.

I knew I was doing important work. I was saving lives, preventing brain death, keeping cardiac output and blood gasses in narrow ranges, treating sepsis, educating families, and comforting patients. But a twelve-hour shift with an ICU patient meant twelve hours in a heightened state of alarm and unwavering vigilance. I struggled to get restful sleep. Daylight peeking around the edges of my blackout blinds was maddening. When I did sleep, I would have nightmares about forgetting to tend to a patient for a whole shift. Working two days and two nights in a row followed by four days off was nice in theory. In reality, it would take a day or two after each shift to recover from sleep deprivation only to begin the process all over again. Ultimately, front line work with unstable patients left me feeling anxious and exhausted.

By this time, my nursing career was in critical condition. Without intervention my career would've met its demise long before its life expectancy of thirty years. Having quickly reached (what I considered to be) the pinnacle of bedside nursing positions, working in ICU nursing was like discovering that the Wizard of Oz was a small man behind the curtain. The idea that I had built up about how fulfilling and exciting it would be, was far from my reality.

The workplace politics that plagued other floors in the hospital were also present in the ICU and drained me of my passion. My career needed as much life support as the patient in the bed in front of me. It felt futile to invest more time, energy, and money into a career I felt limited by, so I continued to show up day after day while fantasizing about a mental health leave of absence.

Emotional exhaustion prohibited me from providing my usual level of attention and care. I started making mistakes that I could not afford for the sake of my patients. As near misses became more common, I could no longer ignore the fact that I needed out of the ICU before I accidentally added an extra decimal point to a critical infusion...again.

I attempted an intervention. Red wine and journal in hand, I reflected on what I really wanted in my life and career. I wrote a list of things I thought would make working feel worthwhile.

- Schedule. Four 10-hour day shifts.
- Money. A six-figure salary.

- Vacation. Six weeks a year.
- Health. To be in the best shape of my life.
- Travel. Once or twice a year. London, Paris, and the Amalfi Coast.
- Family. To have a baby by 35, with or without a partner.

I didn't know what I needed to do to achieve the items on my list, but I had a vision for my life for the first time in a long time. The way I viewed my nursing career shifted from that point forward. I started to make choices that would purposefully change my career trajectory in the direction that I *wanted* instead of following the safe route.

Around this time, a spot opened on the NRT unit council, comprised of nurses, a nurse educator and the nurse manager who met on a monthly basis to make recommendations to improve work-life balance, safety, and patient care. I asked myself, who would take this type of position? The answer was what I aspired to be; someone who didn't play it safe, someone who would risk being visible.

I thought about the head of my Queen's nursing class council who had worked with the World Health Organization in Geneva between semesters. She seemed to always slide into opportunities that I didn't even know existed, and I quietly admired her for it. Joining the unit council seemed like an opportunity that *she* would have acted on, so I applied.

People who know me now would be surprised to find out that this move was out of character. I was the type of student who never raised their hand to ask a question and never stayed behind to chit-chat with the professor. I didn't volunteer for activities that I wouldn't be paid for or that wouldn't be supplemented by some adult beverages. At this point in my life, getting involved in an extracurricular leadership opportunity was very unlike me.

From that *one* decision, *many* doors opened. I got to know the Manager and Educator of my unit better. I had a taste of what it was like to be paid for time spent away from the bedside. I worked toward positive change for my nurse colleagues. Participating in the unit council felt tremendously satisfying, energizing, and not at all like work.

MY NURSING STORY

A year later, I nominated myself for the position of unit council Chair, and voilà! As a relatively novice nurse, I found myself not just a participant, but a leader. I was scared it would be a stretch of my abilities, but it wasn't. I dove in and enjoyed every minute. I planned and led annual team-building days, got a pulse on what the NRT nurses felt they needed, and started to advocate.

Around this time, I was encouraged to apply for a new hospital-wide nursing fellowship. Since I was on a roll applying for leadership-type opportunities that I didn't think I was qualified for, I applied. To my surprise, I was awarded a fellowship! The imposter syndrome in me said I only got a spot because too few other people applied so I attended each meeting feeling a little out of place. Looking back, I know I deserved my spot every bit as much as the nurse sitting next to me.

The fellowship moved me even further away from bedside work toward what I was becoming increasingly passionate about - the well-being of my nursing colleagues. I spent twenty percent of my working hours being mentored toward achieving my goal of building a conference for NRT nurses. The intent of the conference was to learn about common challenges and brainstorm solutions. With a six-month deadline, I took action. I found the contact information for nurse managers and educators from NRT units in hospitals within a 2-hour drive. I made cold calls and sent unsolicited emails. I figured out logistics and very shyly asked the Chief Nursing Officer of the hospital for funding - to which she agreed!

Ultimately, more than 100 nurses and nurse leaders came together for the inaugural conference event which was a near-complete success. My one regret? I charged only $20 a person. In terms of profit, there was none. The low cost to participate and zero profit realized reflected my money beliefs at the time and perhaps the money beliefs of my mentors, as no one encouraged me to charge more.

I continued for a few years in this fashion, taking on leadership opportunities I didn't think I was qualified for as they arose. Despite my feeling that the roles may get me closer to my ideal career goals, I often felt like an imposter. I was doing what I thought someone *else* would do. Not necessarily, what *I* would do. I was growing into the idea of being some sort of leader and change maker, someone with a higher income, but I had a long way to go.

More education

After a few years of contemplation, I applied to a Master's and Nurse Practitioner (NP) program. I was living in alignment with my values: happy, confident, and in the best shape of my life. Going back to school to upgrade my education and build my capacity for leadership seemed like the next logical step.

For all of my personal growth, I still chose my Master's stream in a very safe way. I asked myself, "What would be most secure?" I wasn't sure if I preferred clinical nursing or nursing leadership, or what my job prospects might be. So, I went with the broad choice of a Master's Degree in Nursing and NP certification for more career options.

I also started dating the man who would become my husband. He had just opened his first personal training studio, a business that is now very much *ours*. It was my first exposure to entrepreneurship. My career had been laser-focused on clinical nursing. As far as I was concerned, nurses made money working for big organizations like hospitals and only made as much money as was offered to them.

As a personal trainer, my husband was charging double or triple what I was making an hour without the anxiety of saving lives or the sleep deprivation of shift work. Instead of spending his time and money on a university degree, he had traveled around the world to learn from the most successful fitness experts in his field, and he hired a mentor who helped him crack the entrepreneurship code. He was able to work only a few hours in the morning and a few hours in the evening leaving time in the day to walk his dog, sit leisurely with a double espresso and get his own workouts in.

My eyes were opened to possibilities I didn't even know existed! *His* was the type of life I wanted and the type of money I wanted to make! Why didn't I have any role models for such a life? No one in my social circle was doing what he was doing as a career; charging a fee-for-service and making their own hours. My only role models had been my parents who worked overtime to scrape up enough money for an occasional camping vacation and saving for a rainy day. The saying, "Everything that can go wrong, will" was my money mantra.

What I came to realize was that no amount of overtime, weekend, or holiday nursing shifts could manifest the type of money and schedule I wanted. If I wanted a balanced life that allowed me to enjoy every day, continue to serve people, and make enough money to do more than survive, I couldn't continue in the conventional way I had been taught in school.

My husband taught me that a university education was not the only road to success. Following your passion and being authentic has as much potential or more for success.

I was lucky to have another example of someone following their passion and achieving financial success. My cousin, Zombie boy, was tattooed from head to toe. His ability to be completely himself, to ignore societal norms and advice contrary to *his* vision of living life to the fullest, led others to take notice. He was discovered by a photographer which led to music videos with Lady Gaga and appearing in movies such as *47 Ronan*. He walked the runways of Paris and Milan, was immortalized in bronze and wax statues and even had his likeness modeled into an action figure that he proudly unveiled to our grandmother one Christmas. While his life was tragically cut short by an unfortunate accident, there can be no doubt that he followed his heart. When I think of authenticity embodied, I think of him.

In the last semester of my Master's Degree, I applied for my first Nurse Practitioner position with a former preceptor who owned an Executive Health clinic. Despite knowing the clinic owner, I was intimidated at the prospect. The clinic was located in the most upscale part of Toronto with a very wealthy clientele. Despite secret desires to have abundant amounts of money, I was intimidated by "rich" people, and these were the *super-rich*. I thought they wouldn't want to work with someone like me. After all, how could we relate? Furthermore, I had been warned against Executive Health by another Nurse Practitioner who told horror stories of unrealistic client expectations.

Despite my initial hesitation, their preventative approach to care appealed to me. Having become deeply familiar with the fitness industry and the emerging field of functional medicine, the opportunity to practice in a preventative model aligned me to their mission even if I couldn't relate to having significant financial resources.

I was invited to interview even though the clinic had already put out a contract offer to another student from my class. Lucky for me, the other applicant was slow to accept. The "fit" seemed right and I was offered the position. After some back and forth in contract negotiation, I accepted my first Nurse Practitioner position before the end of my last semester.

One year later, driven by a desire to improve conditions for clients and colleagues, I was offered the position of Clinic Director. After attaining this prestigious position, with prestigious clientele, and a high level of success, you would think I would be pretty satisfied with my career? However, I was still far from aligned with my true self. It turned out that the clinic wasn't as aligned with my values as I had hoped. While they touted a preventative approach, I was run ragged. I had failed to set boundaries and I was virtually on call for the clients and staff. I fell back into old habits and coped by stress eating - and no, I wasn't reaching for a head of broccoli for comfort. Three years into my tenure at the clinic, I had gained thirty pounds on my five-foot two frame. I had sacrificed myself and felt worse than ever.

My true self is a no-nonsense person. I am the friend who will tell you if you have parsley in your teeth or when your make-up looks like it was done by a 5-year-old! My personality may not appeal to everybody, but as a nurse I adapted myself to become a version palatable to most. Only when I started to rediscover and express my authentic self, did I start to feel truly aligned and begin to break through my nursing income barrier.

Realizing that a fancy title and marble-floored office wasn't for me, I started searching for other opportunities. I stumbled upon medical cannabis as an emerging area of practice and took an introductory online course. Then, someone in my network informed me of an opportunity at a new NP-led medical cannabis clinic. I applied and started working part-time from home. For the first time in a long while, I felt like I had discovered a clinical area that I could be passionate about. While I didn't take cannabis myself, I found great satisfaction in the success patients were having with medical cannabis plus I was eliminating the barrier to access many patients faced, helping them get relief from their symptoms that other prescriptions couldn't provide.

The unexpected

In 2019, I was on cloud nine. I was working in a field I loved. My husband and I hit the seven-figure mark in our personal training business and had opened a second gym using a significant chunk of our savings. Becoming pregnant was the final gift that realized many of my dreams. I was looking forward to a maternity leave spent attending mommy groups and writing my first book during my son's naps. Then, the pandemic hit.

Lockdowns for gyms came into effect before the paint dried on our new walls! We kept hearing two more weeks, two more weeks…so, we planned to survive for six months because we thought there was no way the economy would be shut down for that long. We were greatly mistaken! To get by, and keep our business alive, we took on six figures in debt. A year later we lost the shiny new second gym, but the debt was here to stay.

Three months into my maternity leave, I went back to work full-time to support our family because our brick-and-mortar business had consumed our savings. Thank goodness I had a work-from-home position to return to. I didn't touch the book I had been so eager to finish writing and I mourned the loss of postpartum bonding with my new baby.

No longer on-call for executive health clients, and now with a child, I started focusing on offering nursing career coaching and writing as a complement to clinical work, and to supplement our lost income from the gym closures.

When I finally got the energy to look at my writing again, I flipped the book I had been writing upside down. I was determined to create something that would be of *real value* to nurses, beyond just telling my story. I developed the Nursing WISELY framework.

I'm now working in a field of nursing I love and pursuing side projects that energize me. I have multiple streams of income and I feel secure, balanced, rewarded, and free.

The key to success is to first know yourself: what drives you, what you enjoy, and then pursue it in spite of nay-sayers or people giving advice in an area where they have no relevant knowledge. My journey has taught me the following:

- Act authentically and follow my gut instinct.
- Apply for opportunities you're not sure you're suited for, but align with your vision of yourself. Remember that you can learn and grow through them.
- Leave jobs when they no longer feel worthwhile or have nothing left to teach you. You may not always come out on top, but you will have few regrets.

When I reflect on my early career, I know I acted slowly to make career transitions and leaps. I put up with boredom, 3:00 am heartburn, and post-traumatic stress induced by Intensive Care Unit (ICU) nursing. It felt easier to show up for shifts I dreaded than to invest the brain power, time, and money required to make a change.

- A stable pay cheque, benefits, and vacation entitlement were blinders that lulled me into a sense of comfort and stability.

- It was easier to stay in the comfortable nursing position I found right out of school that offered great benefits and pension, but didn't offer joy or support for my basic life needs.

- It was easier to clock in twelve hours with substandard staffing ratios and go home without putting in a grievance form, returning to a never-ending short staffing situation than to put my neck out in the name of patient safety. It was easier to assume someone else would raise my concerns. I risked post-traumatic stress, burn-out, medical errors, patient safety, and, most importantly, my health and happiness.

- I used to feel that pursuing extra education without extra pay was absurd. Why would I work harder for nothing immediately tangible in return? Then, I learned how little I knew and it ignited my passion for lifelong learning.

Now, I am more confident, more in control, and I love where I am in my life and career! The first time I shared my story to a group of peers, I realized I was an outlier, but was respected nonetheless. I knew others must share experiences similar to my own. If your experiences have been similar to mine, I hope you feel less alone.

STOP AND THINK

What take-aways do you have after reading my nursing story?

Who, in your life, demonstrates authenticity?

How would being less worried about the opinions of others change your life?

Early in my career, I started to make decisions about opportunities that I thought *others* would make because they were my models for success. Eventually I realized I couldn't have a career I loved unless I created my own path.

MODULE ONE

CREATING A WORTHWHILE CAREER

"I can't imagine anything more worthwhile than doing what I most love. And they pay me for it."

—Edgar Winter

By the end of Module 1, you will have defined what worthwhile means to you. The module starts with reflection - telling your personal story. You will then define your values, identify your ideal niche in nursing, reverse engineer your ideal career, and set goals to help you move toward it. After completing this module, you will be able to write a clear, strong, statement about what you feel makes your career in nursing worthwhile and set goals based on this statement.

WHAT MAKES NURSING WORTHWHILE?

Feeling that what you are doing is worthwhile inspires motivation, happiness, and fulfillment in a career that can otherwise be challenging and lead to burnout. Understanding what "worthwhile" means to you will lay a foundation for your career and can serve as your guiding compass. Skipping this step may lead you to take opportunities that are not in alignment with your values and could affect your feelings of self-worth. Note that your definition of what is worthwhile may evolve as you gain experiences and knowledge.

Don't confuse what is worthwhile with your "why" or "raison d'être." What is worthwhile is an exchange of time, energy, or money that you find of value. It can be tied to your why, but it doesn't stop there. It is also tied to your needs, self-worth, and your values.

I had a colleague who commuted two hours from rural Ontario to downtown Toronto and back for each 12-hour shift. Rain, sleet, or shine, she would hop in her car, crank some tunes, and beat traffic. From my point of view, nothing was worth that commute time, so I asked her why on earth she would do that to herself?

She told me that the year before, she had bought her dream farmhouse which included chickens, a retired show horse named Gwen, a few fluffy sheep, and expansive crop fields. After nearly three decades in the same unit, she felt it was worthwhile to do the commute until retirement, relishing in the joy of her new homestead in her off hours. It wasn't *my* dream, but she had made hers come true and the commute was just a manageable tradeoff. So, what is worthwhile to you?

There are many pros and cons to nursing as a career. Nursing is full of opportunities to pursue your passions, has decent compensation, and flexibility in geographic location, sectors, and schedules. Special moments in nursing can make the less-than-ideal conditions of nursing feel worthwhile; like witnessing a successful resuscitation or the birth of a healthy baby, receiving words of appreciation from patients, and executing the perfect blood draw. You can often go to bed knowing you made a difference in someone's life. Nursing is also full of challenges: pay inequality, shift work, being run off your feet, understaffing, and witnessing death to name a few. My career in nursing has not always been easy, but it has been worth it.

What I do, and the rewards I get—whether financial or emotional—feel worthwhile to me. It wasn't always that way. I've had dark moments in my career where I felt that continuing in nursing wasn't worthwhile. I've held positions that weren't aligned with my needs or discovered that they didn't offer the opportunities I expected. Through self-reflection, I've been able to get my career back on track.

You may be familiar with Maslow's Hierarchy of Needs,[2] depicted using a pyramid with the most basic needs at the bottom. Needs at the bottom of the pyramid must be met before an individual can be motivated to meet the next higher-level need. At the base are our basic *physiological* needs for survival: things like food, clothing, sleep and shelter. Next are *safety* needs like a job, and social services like medical care and policing. Moving up the pyramid is *psychological* needs, including love and the sense of belonging we get from friends, family and colleagues then *esteem* needs or feelings of accomplishment. At the pinnacle of the pyramid is *self-actualization*—being able to fulfill your highest potential. What makes your career "worthwhile" at any point may depend on your needs in that moment.

Early in my career, the money made nursing worthwhile and fulfilled my physiological and safety needs. I joined my unit council which helped me to feel connected to my nursing colleagues, meeting my need for belonging. I then began climbing the nursing career ladder to fulfill the esteem need by gaining respect, recognition, and freedom. Lastly, here I

---

2 Maslow, A. H. (1954). *Motivation and personality*. New York: Harper and Row.

am working toward self-actualization. To become the most I can be, by helping as many nursing colleagues as I can to also move through their careers toward self-actualization.

Using Maslow's Hierarchy can help you to assess what has motivated you in your career thus far as well as understand where your motivation may go when life throws a curve ball, sending you up or down the pyramid at a moment's notice. Some needs, like food or shelter, are extrinsic (coming from outside). While higher level needs like self-actualization are intrinsic (coming from within). Both are important and should be considered when making decisions about your career.

Your family needing food on the table (extrinsic) can be all the motivation you need to show up for a shift despite nagging back soreness or fatigue. But receiving an unexpected inheritance would require you to connect with a deeper motivation (intrinsic) to continue your career in nursing.

Simon Sinek, author of *Start with Why: How Great Leaders Inspire Everyone to Take Action*, calls this deeper source of motivation your "why." Your "why" is a feeling that compels you even if it requires short-term sacrifice. Your "why" gives your work and career meaning. With a strong enough reason to compel you to continue your nursing career, you wouldn't leave the profession, even if you could. You would find ways to contribute to the field of nursing or the well-being of patients or your community beyond retirement even if it was in a different role, like a committee volunteer.

The questions are: "What makes your career worthwhile, and is it enough to keep you in nursing whether times are good or bad?" Answering these questions requires you to examine your career path up to this point.

Your Story

When I see a patient for an initial assessment of a chronic health condition, I pull out a blank paper and pencil and draw a timeline from birth to the present. Along the timeline we note significant past medical history or stressful events the patient has encountered. Then, I ask, "When was the last time you felt truly healthy?" After a significant pause, the patient often responds, "No one has ever asked me that before. I can't remember when I last felt healthy." When stuck in a chronic negative situation - "I feel bad," the patient can barely recall when they last felt *good*.

Now, back up the timeline and add in significant positive life events: birthdays, vacations, the birth of a child, and so on. Once their memory is flooded with positive memories, the patient is usually able to pinpoint when things changed. Once we have that moment on the timeline, we can identify what changed and what needs to be done to move towards a more positive lifestyle or mindset.

Mapping a career offers a similar journey. In expressing your unique story, you will begin to find your voice. Finding that voice will allow you to discover your individual strengths as a nurse and ultimately to adjust your course toward the positive vision you had when you first embarked on your career.

Early in my career, I started to make decisions about opportunities that I thought *others* would make because they were my models for success. Eventually I realized I couldn't have a career I loved unless I created my own path.

Examining our stories draws on the science of phenomenology, the study of consciousness and the objects of direct experience.[3] Put simply, it is a way of thinking about yourself to uncover your truth.

You need to understand where you've been to truly know where you want to go but, this doesn't mean dwelling on the past or the future. Start by appreciating yourself right now. Meet yourself where you are without judgment. See yourself with grace and compassion. Give yourself respect and approval. From this moment forward, make a vow to quiet criticism

---

3 Van Manen, M. (2014). *Phenomenology of practice*. Walnut Creek, CA: Left Coast Press, Inc.

or let it pass through you so that you can get back to doing the amazing things only you are capable of.

Now set aside your beliefs about:

- Whether you are currently at your best or your worst.
- Whether you are capable or incapable of great things.

Instead, begin with an acknowledgment of where you are in your career, schooling, and private life. You deserve credit for making it this far, no matter the current level of energy in your tank or money in the bank. And, here's a secret: you already know who you want to become. Yes! You already know!

I've always known that I wanted to be a writer. I don't find writing easy, but I enjoy it. I've written blog posts for my businesses for a long time, but publishing a book has always been a dream. The prospect of being a published writer intimidated me—heck it still intimidates me! Despite this, I never lost sight of the vision of holding a physical book that I wrote myself. And, here we are!

A colleague of mine shared that from the age of twenty, she secretly knew she wanted to own a luxury medical spa. The first time she visited one, she left feeling like *that* was her future. Every decision to pursue further education in nursing brought her one step closer to that dream. Now twenty years later, she is a Nurse Practitioner specialized in medical aesthetics and is the owner of two med spas in beautifully renovated old homes. She is living her dream that started with *acknowledging a feeling*.

Let the truth about who you want to be and what you want to do come to the forefront from the place you have been denying it. Ask the person you want to be, to move in and stay. Become aware of your dreams and be honest with yourself about your desires. Let yourself imagine a level of success beyond what you think others may believe is possible for you and what you think is possible for yourself.

Remove the lens of negativity and judgment it's time to put on rose-coloured glasses. You can't hold space for self-doubt and also be able to tell yourself the truth about what you want to become next. Despite what your inner gremlin says—you *can*! You are capable.

Need an example to push through the barrier? Think of yourself as an elephant. Elephants are highly intelligent, strong, and intimidating animals. Yet, many elephants have been tamed to bend to the requests of their human captor. How is this possible?

As a baby, an elephant is easily controlled with a rope around their neck. They learn they are not strong enough to break free and there is a boundary established with the length of their rope. As an adult, despite being strong and capable, one must merely put a rope around the elephant's neck. They will stop moving beyond their imagined barrier despite the reality of being able to snap the rope easily.

As novice nurses, we are smart and eager to learn. We grow up to be strong nurses, but we learn the boundaries of our nursing careers from our professors, clinical instructors, and managers. We don our scrubs and leave a portion of our individual identities behind as we step into the role of "nurse" as defined by our colleges and colleagues. We put patients, outcomes and safety first but ignore ourselves.

As we become more seasoned and we feel a desire that is beyond the norms of the profession, we feel anxiety, guilt, and doubt. We stay put in our careers or follow the well-traveled path paved by more senior nurses. Deviation is not the norm, but *there is no actual barrier* to prevent us from pursuing our dreams.

Go ahead. Try to name the barrier that prevented you from achieving what you truly wanted in your career. You may name your nursing college, saying they have set limiting policies, but I assure you there is always room for evolution, change, and continuous improvement in these policies and you have the ability to affect them.

What if the "barrier" you perceive to be there is not real? What if it is an imaginary rope around your neck, made up of learned behaviour and norms, that is holding you captive. These norms may feel safe, but they will not get you where you long to go. They keep your true desires hostage.

It's time to take off that rope! I'm not kidding. Use your hands to loosen the knot, feel the weight of the cord lifting off your shoulders, and hear the rope dropping to the ground. Take a deep breath, it's time to let your aspirations out into the world so you can do great things!

What do we call a nurse who has rid herself of the imaginary rope that led her to ignore her true self? Authentic.

Authenticity is the secret superpower you will harness and leverage to build a fulfilling and successful career. We will dive deeper into the concept of authenticity in Module 6. Now, it is time to share your story and create your timeline.

The following self-assessment exercise will help you to reflect on where you have been as a first step in deciding where you want to go. Take a moment to concentrate on why you are here on this Earth. It's time to get reacquainted with yourself.

EXERCISE: Draw your career path

1. Get out a pen and paper (we're doing this old school!) and draw a line starting at your birth, extending to present day. Don't be afraid to use a few pieces of paper, lining them up end-to-end for more space.
   - Mark key turning points on the path that brought you to where you are in your life and career. Include both stressful and positive events.
2. What are the underlying themes that define you and your life?
3. When was the last time you felt passionate about your career in nursing? What was it about that time that made it feel worthwhile?
4. If you are not satisfied with your career, what changes do you have to make to bring you back to a point where you can feel your work is worthwhile again? If you are already satisfied, what will keep it that way?
5. If this book is successful in getting you moving in the right direction, where would you like to be?

DEFINE YOUR VALUES

IN MY THIRD YEAR AS Nurse Practitioner, I was earning more money than ever, smashing the financial goal I had set for myself as a novice nurse. Between my full-time contract, part-time employment, private practice, and personal training studio my income was more than healthy—but I wasn't. As my income grew, so did my spending habits. I was experiencing lifestyle creep with an ever-expanding taste for the "finer" things like fancy dinners, lavish vacations, and non-stop online shopping. No matter how much money I made, I always felt poor and insecure because I didn't have a safety net in the bank or own any assets like a home or car.

It was hard for me to imagine a time when I was happy living on just $500 a month but, I knew I was happier as a new grad nurse in 2008 than I was as a high-rolling professional in 2018. Why was that?

Early in my career, I made some excellent money choices. I paid down my student loans, put money into my retirement savings, and relished a Friday pizza night as a rare special occasion. Meanwhile, in 2018 I was racking up credit card debt and eating out almost every meal (with a waistline to show for it). New, expensive experiences were starting to feel like a source of stress instead of excitement leading me to stop spending quality time with friends and family because I was so busy trying to fit more work hours into my week. The things I valued above money, including friends, family, and my health, were suffering.

I was living out of alignment with my values. I had to stop the roller coaster of spending what I earned, and get back to basics.

I downloaded budgeting software that connected to my bank accounts and did a deep dive into where my money was going. I kept an eye on it every day for a month. Soon, I had cut my expenses in half, resumed saving and started to feel like my old self.

Many coaching clients come to me with a similar dilemma. They are successful on paper but feel something is off. They can't always put their finger on it, but as we work together, we discover that they are living out of alignment with their values.

Values are the fundamental beliefs that guide or motivate our attitudes or actions. They guide your decisions and are a marker for whether your life is turning out the way you want it to.

When you don't feel good about your life, there's a good chance that you're doing things out of alignment with your values. Likewise, when things are going well and you're excited about life, there's a good chance you're living in alignment with your values. So, making a conscious effort to identify your values is important as you set goals and build your nursing career.

At times, values may compete. You can't always "have-it-all" and so we also need to be able to understand our priorities when it comes to our values. A job may offer high job security, but low pay. You will have to decide what is more important. Knowing what you care about in advance will make decision-making easier.

I value money, but not at the expense of time with family and friends. I value independence, but not at the expense of loneliness. I value helping others, but not at the expense of my health.

To identify your values, think of the times when you were happiest, most proud, fulfilled, or satisfied. What were you doing? Who were you with? What other factors contributed? Try to identify why those experiences were most important and memorable. Here are some examples of values to get you started:

Accountability	Exploration	Preparedness
Achievement	Fairness	Professionalism
Adventurousness	Faith	Prudence
Altruism	Family	Quality
Ambition	Fitness	Reliability
Balance	Freedom	Resourcefulness
Belonging	Fun	Restraint
Calmness	Generosity	Results
Challenge	Goodness	Security
Clear-mindedness	Grace	Self-actualization
Community	Growth	Self-control
Compassion	Happiness	Selflessness
Competitiveness	Hard Work	Self-reliance
Consistency	Health	Simplicity
Control	Honesty	Soundness
Cooperation	Humility	Spontaneity
Correctness	Independence	Stability
Creativity	Intelligence	Status
Curiosity	Intuition	Strength
Decisiveness	Joy	Structure
Dependability	Justice	Success
Determination	Leadership	Support
Diligence	Legacy	Teamwork
Discipline	Love	Thoroughness
Discretion	Loyalty	Thoughtfulness
Diversity	Making a difference	Timeliness
Effectiveness	Mastery	Trustworthiness
Efficiency	Money	Truth-seeking
Empathy	Openness	Understanding
Enjoyment	Order	Uniqueness
Equality	Originality	Unity
Excellence	Perfection	Usefulness
Excitement	Positivity	Vision
Expertise	Practicality	Vitality

Values are fairly stable, but as you grow in life they can change. Revisiting your values periodically, especially when you are feeling low, anxious, or otherwise unhappy can help get you back on track. Knowing your values helps you to keep in touch with who you are and who you want to be. Let these values guide you to creating a worthwhile career.

EXERCISE: Know your values

1. Think of a time when you were living in alignment with your values. How did it feel?
2. Think of a time when you were living out of alignment with your values. How did it feel? How did you turn it around?
3. Write down your top 12 values. Then, narrow the list to your top 6. Then, to your top 3. These are your guiding values. Keep these in mind as you move forward in this book.

IDENTIFY YOUR NICHE

"Nursing" is a broad title. It represents nurses working:

- with babies, teens, adults, seniors,
- in a community,
- in a prison,
- in a hospital,
- in an office,
- in management, education or research,
- in oncology, cardiology, or neurology,
- with a college diploma, bachelor's degree, master's degree, doctorate,
- creating art or heading nursing magazines,
- creating policy,
- writing textbooks or developing technology,
- in-person doing cosmetic dermatology and fillers,
- working remotely via telemedicine,
- working up north in the Arctic, out of helicopters, or on a cruise ship, and
- in health systems locally, nationally, or globally.

You can see the many opportunities that are available in a nursing career, but you can't be a master of them all.

It is difficult to be an expert neonatal nurse and gerontology nurse at the same time (although I'm sure it's possible if that is your idea of the perfect career!). Preemies and seniors both have basic human needs requiring expert nursing care, but the similarities end there. You can have transferable skills working with the two populations, e.g., good interpersonal skills and attention to detail, but will need to understand different medications, dosing, and pharmacokinetics for the premature versus mature body.

As a nurse, you are equipped to learn to care for any population you prefer, but you have to be honest with yourself about your preferences to come to that decision. Get over the guilty feeling that specializing will cut off your ability to care for absolutely *everybody*.

It's *ok* to have patient population preferences. You can love and value all human beings at every stage of life, but not give direct patient care to them all in your career. Given the opportunity to choose to work with preemies or palliative patients who would you work with? You likely have a preference and are naturally more skilled at working with one population over the other. Maybe you prefer to work away from the bedside. That's okay too.

Few people know exactly what they love and pursue it. Some know what they love and think it's unattainable. Many have no idea and plod along in denial, avoiding examining their preferences or making a choice at all. I've been each of these persons at different points in my career.

In order to do anything meaningful and fulfilling it's important to get specific. If you love being a generalist, then so be it. Own it and give yourself the title: [*insert your name here*] the Expert Generalist Nurse!

When I was employed in the Nursing Resource Team (NRT) at a major teaching hospital there was no bigger definition of a generalist nurse than being able to go from cardiology one day, to neurology the next. I learned a lot and hoped I'd find one area in the hospital that was for me, but I never found that one special unit I wanted to call home. I had to admit to myself that despite the security of hospital employment, it wasn't for me long-term. I had to admit to myself I wanted my career to be specialized and then had to drill down to figure out what that specialization meant for me.

You are unique and your career should be too. There is a space and need for every nurse. Some spaces already exist and others have yet to be created.

A "niche" is a position or activity that particularly suits somebody's talents and personality. It's an area of practice that you can make your own and a patient population or care need you can meet. By choosing a niche, you can focus your professional growth and build your career around an area of practice that you are passionate about.

For example, one of my mentors wrote her Ph.D. thesis on pet therapy! How is that for a niche? She combined her love of mental health nursing with her love of animals. She now dabbles in several areas, including: academics, Nurse Practitioner Practice in Medical Cannabis and Sexual Health, and Cognitive Behavioural Therapy. Imagine how awesome would it be if she pulled together *all* of her expertise and passions? Perhaps a niche pet therapy business for those who have experienced sexual trauma!

The goal of Module 1 is to help you identify your passions and areas of expertise, so that you can pick a niche and create your ideal career. Earlier, we explored your nursing career story to get back to your nursing roots, then we talked about values. Now, we need to get specific.

The exercise questions in this section will help you to think about, and describe, the types of patients or clinical conditions or work environments that bring you the most joy. What leaves you with the most satisfaction at the end of the day? What allows you to balance work and the rest of your life? What are you excited to continue learning about, and who are you excited to learn from?

These are not easy questions. Perhaps you feel blocked because the answers run counter to the values that nursing school taught or perhaps your ego is getting in the way. At times, my ego is my biggest enemy. It wants to protect me from failure, disappointment, and pain, and being stubborn doesn't help! So, how did I overcome the resistance?

Well, it took me nearly *ten years* to admit where my passion lay. I started my career by experiencing as many different roles and populations as possible. Every time a new opportunity presented itself, I took it. I became an expert generalist, but it was not by design. I knew a little bit about a lot of things but I never found my home in a specific area of nursing because I was dabbling in areas that I already knew deep down weren't my passion.

The pattern of denying my true interests started as a nursing student. For my undergraduate consolidation, I ignored my lifelong disdain for cold weather and applied for Queens' Moose Factory (renamed in 2020 to the Weeneebayko Program). Haven't heard of Moose Factory? That's because it is so remote you need to travel north using air, boat and an ice road depending on the time of year!

I had no particular interest in Northern nursing and no intention to build a career in the North yet I left my university housemates behind and hopped on a single-engine aircraft to live in a remote community for three months where the *average* temperature was -40 Celsius/Fahrenheit! It was so cold that steam heat was distributed through the community via a pipe system where you would expect there to be electricity lines.

It *was* a unique experience that I will never forget. I am forever grateful for opening my eyes to the realities of remote living (hello $10 overripe bananas) and the lived realities of Canadian history that are not taught in school (I can't believe I had never heard of residential schools). However, the guilt of wondering if I took the spot of another nursing student who had a passion for Northern nursing and would have gone on to serve that community, plagued me for several years.

As I've shared, my first nursing position following graduation was working at a major urban teaching hospital as part of the Nursing Resource Team for medical, surgical and step-down units, day surgery, the emergency department, and intensive care units. I saw it all and kept my mind open to settling down in one unit. Several years later, I was still with the NRT and no closer to identifying my ideal bedside position.

I made lateral moves and bulked up my resume. I took leadership opportunities, including working in corporate nursing and on Ministry of Health funded projects. I participated in the unit and hospital-wide nursing councils, and completed a nursing fellowship. I went to networking events for future healthcare leaders. I chased many "shiny objects" but lacked a broad view of my future possibilities and for all of my experience, I didn't earn more money.

In Ontario, there wasn't a bonus for specialization. I felt like I was going in circles. Each move felt like procrastination, pushing down my career desires and making excuses for why I couldn't pursue the things I wanted. The real reason I couldn't nail down a patient population to work with was because I was too busy avoiding opportunities in psychiatric and mental health nursing—the areas I truly felt pulled toward. I was denying what I already knew, and resisting where my actions were propelling me.

But there were positives. I encountered formal and informal nursing mentors who I admired. They filled my head with crazy ideas like being an emerging leader, when I still saw myself as a novice nurse. They emphasized the importance of using my full name and title, the need to cultivate unshakable confidence, inspired an ability to create new opportunities for myself, and underlined the importance of career planning.

After a dizzying start to my career, I finally got honest with myself. By reflecting on all of the experiences I had, I uncovered what truly made me feel happy and fulfilled—connecting with other nurses to solve problems and improve their lives; mental health nursing for nurses!

On the nursing unit council, we worked to solve issues at the individual and unit levels. In the nursing professional practice council, we worked to solve issues at an organizational level. Creating the NRT conference gave me the opportunity to see the nurses, nurse educators, and nurse leaders working together, using appreciative inquiry to learn from each other, and taking lessons back to their respective organizations. As a Nurse Practitioner in independent practice, I made myself publicly available to nursing colleagues through an online forum that grew to over 1,000 members. These colleagues naturally reached out for career and business help and the flow of that advice came naturally to me.

I know that serving other nurses is my calling because these are the experiences that energize me. Conversations with other nurses on how to get that job they're looking for, or what education they should pursue to get to the next step in their career don't feel like work, they feel fulfilling and worthwhile.

The entire profession of nursing revolves around the values of helping, giving, and altruism. Admitting that I preferred caring for colleagues over caring for patients (especially as a Nurse Practitioner who had dedicated her career and education to caring for *patients*) was tough for me.

My niche is *nurse career empowerment*, and my ideal clients are nurses at any stage in their career looking for their place in nursing.

Early on, I spent my career "going wide." I prided myself on gaining broad experience but success comes when you stop going broad and go deep into the area that brings joy and excitement. Yes, career coaching for nursing existed, but *me* as a nursing career coach – that possibility hadn't emerged but I knew it would. I knew this was my path.

I was finally able to uncover and accept a recurring theme—the thing I came back to in my mind over and over—what I felt my heart was pulling me toward. All of a sudden, the pull to write, specifically about nursing careers, money, and mental health made sense! The pull to build up my nursing colleagues, and help them step into their ideal careers became an attainable goal.

I started collecting stories from colleagues, reaching out to other nurse entrepreneurs to learn from their experiences. Hastily written sentences and paragraphs typed into the notes program in my phone—recorded musings on nursing, career, and life that were divinely downloaded to my brain while standing on a crowded subway platform, on brief lunch breaks or in stolen moments between patients—came together.

I couldn't ignore my desire to go deep, to stop pretending I wanted to "do it all." Instead, I recognized there were plenty of other nurses who could replace me in my other roles and they would do it with more grace, ease, and pleasure than I could ever muster! Now, it's your turn. Take time to reflect, and then take action, with the exercise below.

EXERCISE: What is your ideal niche?

1. What area of your nursing practice or personal life brings you the most joy? What type of problems do you enjoy solving? If you're not sure, do a quick internet search of nursing areas of practice. If you come across something that piques your interest, write it down.

2. Reach out to nurses in your circle to ask them about their careers and areas of practice. Ask what they enjoy and don't enjoy, or the best and worst parts of their jobs. See if any of their experiences resonate with you.

   - Go a step further. Identify nurses who are working in areas you are interested in. Reach out on a social platform (LinkedIn or Facebook) or ask a colleague to introduce you. Offer to pay for their time to consult them about their career - invite them to become part of your network as you work toward obtaining your ideal career.

3. Imagine your ideal client and get specific. Write down as many details as you can. What is the client's age, sex, gender, and marital status? Where do they live? Do they have children or pets? What do they do for a living?

4. What problem will you solve for them? What are their pain points?

5. How would you like to help them?

REVERSE ENGINEERING YOUR NURSING CAREER

WHEN YOU CHANGE A WOUND dressing applied by another nurse, how do you go about it? Do you quickly rip it off, apply whatever you have on hand and then move on? Do you read the previous nurse's note to see the description of the wound and the materials used? Or, is there another way?

I promise you will ensure a better outcome for the patient, if you work backward and pay attention as you disassemble each layer of the dressing. Observing each step, in reverse, that the previous nurse would have taken to successfully dress the wound. Then, once the wound bed is exposed, you decide for *yourself* how best to go about dressing it. Will you add a new cutting-edge dressing or stick with the tried and true? Once you have an end goal in mind, you can plan step-by-step actions, put them in place and be ready to improvise if needed to meet the best possible outcome.

Every nursing plan needs a desired outcome, but no two plans need to be alike. While there may be best practices, lived experience should also come into play. Similarly, we can reverse engineer our careers, but no two careers need be exactly alike. I encourage you to look at the paths of others who have had a nursing career you would like to have, and then envision your path. Ask yourself, "Looking back from retirement, what does a successful career look like for me?"

When you initially make a career plan, you may choose the simplest route:

A. Get the letters behind my name.
B. Get a job with a pension.
C. Retire at age 55.

While the simple route offers a straight path, it may not offer the most fulfilling experience. Also, a lack of proper planning may not leave you with enough money to retire with! Nursing WISELY will help you to make a plan that checks all the boxes on your career list, including being personally fulfilling.

Would you rather fly over Paris on your way to Italy or do a 24-hour stopover and indulge in a fresh croissant and some macarons?

Some professionals describe their careers as jumping from lily pad to lily pad, others feel it's more like a long and winding road. I have *never* heard anyone describe their careers as a straight line to the "top." You may pause to have children, or there may come a time when you are forced to take a leave due to injury or to mourn a loss. You may receive a unique opportunity to change direction or need to pivot when the wind is knocked out of your sails. Make a plan, but stay flexible so that you can have a quality of life on your journey to your dream career.

This module isn't about outlining the steps to your dream career that you *have* to take, rather it's about crafting a journey you *want* to take.

I also encourage you to reverse engineer your retirement fund. Sit down with a financial advisor and figure out how much you need in savings, to have the type of retirement that you want. If you're currently deep in debt you need to know your options; from making a budget to declaring bankruptcy and rebuilding from zero. You can't go through your career blind to its financial destination.

If there is anything that going through a pandemic and working in healthcare can teach you, it is that an abundant life does not mean dying with the biggest house and the most toys. A rich career is rich in time, family and friends, knowledge, experience, collegiality, and legacy.

Imagine your retirement. How many zeros are on your bank balance and can you visualize sitting by the pool in Boca Raton, sipping piña coladas and playing cards with Marge? Who is part of your social circle? What memories will you have created, and what on earth you will do with your newfound free time! After all, as many of my patients have found out, retirement is a tough transition if you don't have anything worthwhile to occupy your time. If you aren't able to find happiness in your everyday life while working, it is not suddenly going to change when you retire. Further, if you don't use it, you lose it. This applies not only to time and money but also to your brain's ability to learn and grow. If you retire early with nothing to stimulate your brain you are more likely to develop dementia than if you retire after 65.[4] How are you going to keep those brain cells happy and healthy? Perhaps through lifelong learning?

While having a plan is key, there are unpredictable events in life. You can't plan when you will fall in love, have children, lose a parent, encounter a pandemic, and so on. So, give yourself permission to have a non-linear path.

You also can't know what you *don't know* when designing your dream career. What you think your dream career is today, may change in five years and again in ten years. That's ok! Revisiting and reviewing the plan on a regular basis is needed.

What if you achieve your goals earlier than expected?

When I graduated from undergraduate studies, I thought I would one day pursue a master's degree and become a Nurse Practitioner. When I met that goal just eight short years later, with a lot of my career still ahead of me, I needed a new goal. Similar to when I graduated from my undergraduate program, the landscape that appeared after becoming a Nurse Practitioner was vastly different from what I had envisioned. My course had to be steered with more precision to find the right path.

What about when things don't go your way?

When the 2020 pandemic shut down non-essential businesses, I had to shut down my personal training business. A good friend also had to close her medical aesthetics business. We both coped financially by taking out

---

4 Sundström, A., Rönnlund, M., & Josefsson, M. (2020). A nationwide Swedish study of age at retirement and dementia risk. *International Journal of Geriatric Psychiatry*, 35(10), 1243-1249.

business loans, doubling down on nurturing our clients, and taking the opportunity to pause and reflect. We streamlined our systems, focused on adding value and eliminated waste.

With the extra time, my friend was able to do an in-depth review her income from the previous year. She learned that the bulk of her income came from neurotoxin treatments. When she reopened her business, she improved her bottom line by focusing on attracting clients looking for neurotoxins and less on other treatments like laser therapy.

Don't be discouraged if you find the path you envisioned is not exactly the one that plays out in the real world. Stop and reassess. Reimagine and renew your goals. Consider dropping goals that are taking up a lot of time, but don't have the promise of a big payout. In this way, you will always have something exciting ahead and will be less stressed in the moment.

You aren't reading this book by chance. You have set yourself on a path toward professional and personal growth. You have taken a step to invest in your future. You believe there is something more for you than what you have experienced so far. Take a minute and thank yourself for investing in your future happiness by learning to shape your future WISELY.

You may have had trouble focusing on your goals in the past. They may have seemed unattainable as you floundered about chasing shiny objects, or perhaps trial and error was returning you to where you started. The intent of this module has been to help you get clear on your vision and plan so that you are able to channel your efforts enabling you to impact lives in the unique way only you can do best.

Exercise: Imagining the future

1. Write about your ideal day three years from now. Use all your senses – close your eyes, what do you see, what do you feel, what do you smell? Where are you? Who are you with? What are you wearing? What does it feel like? How are you going to spend your day?

2. Go back to the career path you drew earlier in this module and extend it to ten years from now.
    a. Where do you think you'll be in ten years if nothing changes?
    b. Where would you like to be in ten years based on your values and interests?
    c. Work backward and fill in the steps on your career path that would make your future a reality.

3. Look even further down the path, what does retirement look like? How are you keeping yourself happy, healthy, and engaged? Again, work backward and put in your steps to retirement.

4. Have a conversation with yourself and answer:
    a. Who was I?
    b. Who am I?
    c. Who will I be?

SET WORTHWHILE GOALS

DID YOU RENEW YOUR NURSING license this year? If so, you may be familiar with goal setting and, you may think you hate it!

Where I live, annual "Quality Assurance" self-reflection and goal setting is a requirement for nursing license renewal. Many nurses resent it. A bigger shame is how many don't bother to complete it, hoping not to get a letter in the mail for a review! Instead of being seen as an opportunity for professional development and a launching point for a happy, healthy career, Quality Assurance is positioned by the College of Nurses of Ontario [5] as assuring the public of nurses' commitment to continuing competence by continually improving their nursing practice.

Did that description compel you to whip out your leather-bound journal and monogrammed pen to get to work? Me neither! Learning goals based on "assured commitment?" Boring! I want to know what is in it for me?

Pay close attention. Here's what your Nursing College failed to tell you about *why* you need to create and revisit your goals on a yearly (at a minimum) basis.

Maybe you set goals in the past and then failed to meet them. This may have led you to believe goal setting is a pointless exercise. I'm telling you it is not - success is often the product of multiple failures. I remind my clients who are attempting to quit smoking that it takes, on average, 7-14 attempts to successfully quit. This will hold true with most efforts to change and to reach a goal. Attempts are not failures. The only true failure is to not try in the first place.

Our brains are powerfully wired for efficiency. Unlearning old patterns and building new neural connections takes commitment and persistence.

---

5 College of Nurses of Ontario. (n.d.). MyQA - Quality Assurance for Nurses. Retrieved March 31, 2023, from https://www.cno.org/en/myqa/.

Watching my son repeatedly get up on his feet while learning to walk reminded me of the persistence it takes to make big shifts. We were all babies once and our egos didn't stop us from repeated attempts. It was no big deal. As an adult, most of us have forgotten how to get back up. We ignore the power of resilience, created the idea of failure, labelling it negative instead of positive. Now is the time to bring back the spirit of your 2-year-old self as you set and attempt to meet your goals.

Why does change require so many attempts?

First, our brains love simplicity. The path of least resistance is the name of the game. Changing a habit requires your body and mind to move out of their usual programming and into entirely new patterns. Your brain adds new circuitry as it learns new things and prunes away old circuitry for efficiency. Circuits are strengthened when they seem to be serving a purpose, whether positive or negative. A habit or behaviour that no longer serves you is dysfunctional but the brain doesn't know that, unless you work to change it.

If you want to achieve something different from what you have now, your brain will need direction. Setting a goal is the first step. Then, to rewire your brain, you have to take repeated steps toward your goal over time. As you move forward, you'll start to lay down new wiring and prune away the old. What if you maintain the status quo? With inaction your brain will prune relentlessly in the name of efficiency, deepening the connection to the programming you don't want to keep.

Think of yourself as a loving nurse and your brain as a pediatric patient. Give your patient rich nutrition, hydration, and some sunshine. Keep your patient away from deadly hazards and negativity that will put them in danger. Speak nicely to that youngster and cheer them on! These efforts will result in growth.

The next step concerns hormones and biochemical patterns. Hormones are the body's messengers. They send signals to our cells telling them how to react in any given moment.

Consider this example. I see failure as a positive and not a negative. But that's not how it started. I had to teach my body to react in a way consistent with this view of the world. In the wild, failure means being eaten by a predator. When threatened, your hormones tell your body to release sugar into the bloodstream so that you can use it for energy to run away or fight. In our modern society, failure means much less and oftentimes is not a failure at all. Rarely does it require a huge mobilization of glucose. Sometimes we even fail up - getting promoted despite mediocre work.

STOP AND THINK
Think of the last time you failed. How did it make you feel? Did you survive it?

Instead of sending paralyzing danger signals when you come up against failure, recognize your thoughts and feelings and get *curious*. Curiosity will send out a different type of hormone and start a whole other cascade that will keep you in motion. There is nothing wrong with trying and failing, it is my preference over inaction and stagnation.

Humans grow through trial and error. We are motivated to move. Our hormones and cellular signaling favour movement. But our society has evolved in a manner that requires us to move less and less. Our physiology hasn't caught up to the new world. Anxiety is often a manifestation of inaction. Our bodies and minds have energy but nowhere to put it. Once you open up and get started, anxiety melts away therefore our goal setting has to satisfy our most basic to most complex needs.

How do we set goals?

There are many methods, but which one is the best? The best tool—like the best diet—is the one we will actually stick to.

Setting goals can be exciting as you envision the outcomes, but once the excitement wears off, you will need a compelling reason to persist toward your goals every day. The following method connects to your emotions and to your greater purpose to make your goals feel worthwhile.

SMART goals

Let's start with goal setting basics. A SMART goal is specific, measurable, attainable, relevant, and time-limited. This is the type of goal you might be required to create for a nursing school placement or yearly professional learning plan.

As health care practitioners, we gain a lot of tools in our tool chest, but we often don't use them. Our tool chests get dusty and the tools rust. Take this opportunity to polish up a tool you may already be using.

Identifying a goal

My client Jenny worked in hospital at the bedside when she suffered a devastating back injury while transferring a patient from bed to stretcher. The injury left her bedridden most hours of the day. Prior to her injury she felt guilty because she loved her career and her family, but never figured out how to balance the two. Now that she faced the possibility of never being able to return to bedside work, she knew she needed to identify a way to support her family while working from home. She had a desire to maintain her nursing license and work hours that allowed her to spend more time with her family. There were a couple of ways Jenny could go about setting her goal.

Example #1: Simplest route from A to B. Become employed remotely as a nurse.

Example #2: Investigate employment and self-employment opportunities in-line with her niche, interests and values.

STOP AND THINK

Which of these goals will be more compelling and have a bigger impact? Why? The more personal the topic, the more motivating the goal.

Specific

Let's continue with the example of the goal of earning a living remotely (the topic), now it's time to get specific. Jenny heard from another colleague that they were earning more as a health coach while working fewer hours than in a traditional nursing role. Jenny always enjoyed the health teaching she did with patients, so she identified virtual nurse health coaching as the type of remote work she wanted to pursue.

Measurable

Add numbers or outcomes to your goal. For example: create a business plan in one week, gain your first client in one month, book 20 client hours a week in 4 months.

Attainable

The most common error in setting goals is not being clear and honest about what you want to achieve and therefore aiming too low. Aiming too low can make your goals attainable, but will not significantly increase your capabilities or create impact. Set the bar high enough to make it worth it to do the work, even if it's tempting to grab the low-hanging fruit and get the serotonin boost.

In our example, it might have been easy for Jenny to simply read a book about nurse health coaching, but to take a course with mentorship and business training will be more effective and more likely to guarantee success.

Relevant

If Jenny wanted to build a career in nurse health coaching, but had chosen a goal to learn about electrocardiograms, she would have been off the mark. At every stage of goal setting, remind yourself of the bigger vision and ask, is this getting me closer to the life and career I want?

Time-limited

Goals without deadlines are just dreams. Hold yourself accountable by setting a reasonable timeline to complete your goal.

SMART goal setting for Jenny would have been, "To identify and complete a nurse health coaching course, with business and practice mentorship included, within three months. Obtain my first client within four months."

Short-term and long-term goals

A long-term goal is an overarching goal that you will meet by completing smaller short-term goals. Short-term goals break down big ambitions into manageable parts. We become experts skill by skill, concept by concept, assessment by assessment, diagnosis by diagnosis, plan by plan, intervention by intervention, and outcome by outcome. One patient at a time.

From our example, the goal of identifying and completing a course is a decent example of a short-term goal. It's relatively safe because we haven't had to make any significant intervention or change.

Increased knowledge is nice, but wouldn't it be much more compelling to be able to say you helped improve thousands of lives over the next ten years? Yes? Then, that would be your long-term goal.

Value-based goals

Let's take goal setting up another notch.

By being specific about what is most important to you, you can commit to your goals at a deeper level. Earlier in this module you identified your values. Values are the compass, with goals as the destination.

STOP AND THINK

On a scale of zero (not at all) to ten (completely), consider how you are living in accordance to the three core values you previously identified.

Once you know your values and how much you are living in alignment with them, you can apply them to your goals. Ask yourself,

- If I was living in alignment with my values, what would I want my life to be like?
- If I was feeling 25% more in line with my values, what would I be doing differently?
- What small thing can I do today to start living according to my values?

Work the answers to these questions into your goals to be sure to be working on the things that are most important to you.

Infinite goals

You may be familiar with the concept of a multiverse. The idea is that multiple possible futures may exist. While this sounds far-fetched, philosophers and physicists are exploring the concept. Likewise, I find using an infinite, rather than finite lens, to be the most compelling part of goal setting.

For example, I have a Master's degree and a successful career. Sometimes I find myself saying I need a Ph.D. I would love to teach at a university level and be a professor to influence fledgling and experienced nurses. I would also love to dabble in nursing and health politics to create change for a female-dominated profession founded in the dark ages, bringing it up to 21st-century standards of gender parity in pay, autonomy, and respect.

Instead of looking at the obvious option of applying to a doctoral program, I step back and ask, "If I want a Ph.D., what are all the possible timelines and avenues to get one?"

I can imagine the options for locations, schools, lengths of time, and costs. Can I achieve it fast? What if I achieve it slowly? Or, not at all? I consider the possible realities of where I would live while completing a Ph.D. such as locked in a library on campus, in a log cabin with good wifi, or in a downsized condo near a university. I ask, what are the outcomes I see myself achieving after earning a Ph.D.? Professorship? Research? In rooms with clients, students, or government officials? Every time I do this activity, I remind myself that there are so many *potential* futures and they are all *possible*!

Of course, I also come to realize I don't *need* a Ph.D. to reach my desired outcomes. I can multiply my reach by acting more and delivering more messages publicly. I can research what I am passionate about and share what I have learned without the approval and censorship of a committee. I know enough. I am doing enough. I have lessons to share and a curriculum in mind to teach.

It is human nature to look towards the next career rung and take the next most logical step. It takes some real self-exploration to go against the well-trodden path and trail blaze.

Ok, it's clear...I don't *need* a Ph.D., but I still *want* one. I have the desire to do the things that would earn me this degree and a desire for the things that would come from earning one. When I looked closer at my career goal of earning a Ph.D. I realized there are multiple ways to achieve this goal.

Multiple ways? Really? Yes! But without doing the exercise of envisioning multiple possible futures I wouldn't have realized this. Here are two possible paths:

Route A: I could take the traditional route of applying to a program, paying a fee and spending five years researching a topic that my supervisor is passionate about, write and defend a thesis, get my cap and gown and cross the stage to accept a Ph.D. Then, get a professorship and grow the profession.

Route B: Pursue professional excellence, expand my reach, promote the profession, and invite others to expand their minds to personal and professional possibilities. Write a book! Specifically, spend as much or as little time as necessary to write a book I am passionate about that I know will propel the profession forward. Get this book in the hands of nursing students, nurses, and nursing leaders. Show up! Grow the profession organically beyond just one nursing class at a time. Get nominated for an honorary Ph.D. at one of my former Alma Maters (looking at you Queen's University). Get my cap and gown and cross the stage to accept a Ph.D. to the delight of many who feel they contributed to my success as I contributed to theirs!

Can you tell which scenario I found more compelling? My goal changed very quickly from getting a Ph.D. to getting an *honorary* Ph.D.

Realizing that there is more than one way to reach a goal is valuable. Making the decision to work to earn an honorary Ph.D. is the goal I like best. I'm now taking action to make it happen and if I fail in my mission, I will have thoroughly enjoyed the journey!

Worthwhile

Once you have your goals, ask yourself are they worthwhile? Are they worth your time, effort, and money? Is your inner voice shouting, "Heck yeah!" or "Hell, no!" Or, is it in defensive mode saying, "None of your business!" To which I would reply, "It is absolutely your business so stop fooling yourself!"

When times get tough you may feel your goals are not worthwhile. This may be a symptom of fatigue, anxiety, depression, imposter syndrome, or burnout. You may need help to decide if those feelings are worthwhile sacrifices. Seek an outside opinion of a mental health professional. We'll touch base on mental health in Module 6.

EXERCISE: Be playful with your goals

This is your chance to think of all the possibilities to create a career that you truly enjoy.

1. What are the multiple ways, including possible paths, to achieve your goals?
2. What are the *outcomes* you're looking to achieve? How can you achieve those outcomes? Consider traditional vs. non-traditional pathways.
3. Does this exercise expand your view of your world and your future? How so?
4. Have you changed your goals? What new goals have you set?
5. How will you feel once you achieve your goals?
6. Create three SMART goals for your nursing career.
7. Are they worthwhile?

ACHIEVE YOUR GOALS

Congratulations! You now have worthwhile goals that excite you! What comes next?

Think about how you learned to become a nurse. Did you enter the doors of your nursing school and *poof* nurse? No, the curriculum was broken down into manageable chunks. Let's do what we know works, and break your goals into achievable steps.

The truth is that most people assume successful people are doing all the things at once, but most really successful people actually only pursue one or two goals at a time. As you build your goal achievement muscle you can add more to the list.

Start with either the goal that excites you most, is easiest to achieve, or will make the biggest impression on your career.

Planning for success

When you learn a new skill, you break it down into manageable components. To make a bed, you need to collect the bedding, remove the previous bedding, then put on the sheets starting with the bottom sheet first. This can get more complex and take a bit longer when there is a patient in the bed, even longer when there has been a code brown, and even more so when that patient is in the ICU and their blood pressure can tank with a mere 10-degree turn.

Whether a goal is simple or complex, breaking it down in a logical order can help take away the intimidation factor and get you on your way.

STOP AND THINK

Break down your goals into the steps you need to take to accomplish them. Then, put them on a timeline to understand how long each goal may take.

I created the following Gantt chart for my application to the "Nurses for Tomorrow" fellowship with my overarching goal to create a conference for the Nursing Resource Teams. A Gantt chart is a standard project management planning tool, but they don't teach it in nursing school!

	20-Sep	27-Sep	4-Oct	11-Oct	18-Oct	25-Oct	1-Nov	8-Nov	15-Nov	22-Nov	29-Nov	6-Dec	13-Dec	20-Dec	27-Dec	3-Jan	10-Jan	17-Jan	24-Jan	31-Jan	7-Feb	14-Feb	21-Feb	28-Feb	6-Mar	13-Mar	20-Mar	27-Mar
Fellowship Workshop																												
Biweekly Mentorship																												
Monthly Manager Update																												
Unit Council																												
Conference Committee																												
Environment Scan/Site																												
Book Venue																												
Call for Abstracts																												
Advertising/Web Site																												
Budget Projection																												
Develop Forum Agenda																												
Develop Printed Material																												
Online Registration																												
Conference																												
Final Write Up																												

Down the left-hand side are the tasks that needed to be completed. Across the top, each week is labeled. Where the two intersect, a square is shaded to indicate when to work on each task. You can easily look at the date and see what you're supposed to be working on that week.

Each task was further broken down into smaller tasks that I could check off one by one. For example, the environment scan was broken down into the following:

- identifying hospitals with NRTs to invite
- getting contact information of NRT nurse managers and educators
- writing an e-mail and/or making a phone call to each person identified to gauge interest
- polling via an electronic survey to determine best dates, price, topics, and format
- identifying a theme from the survey

Celebrating success

If you ever needed an excuse to celebrate, achieving a goal is a reason to do it! What did you do after your final nursing exam? Did you grab a celebratory drink, take a vacation, or buy a new pair of scrubs? Every goal achieved is a milestone. Plan ahead. What are you going to do to mark achievement of your goal(s)?

Revisiting goals

When I turned twenty, I created a bucket list of 100 goals. To get my first nursing job, to complete a master's degree, to become a nurse practitioner, to travel to ten countries, to have a family, to publish a book, and so on. All of my goals started off as ideas written on paper and, over the years, have been gradually checked off. When I look at goals set all those years ago, I can't remember exactly who I was at the time, but I surprise myself when I've checked things off that I didn't even remember having written down! Were it not for goal setting I would not be where I am or who I am today.

Now, 100 goals is *a lot* of goals. Too many for one year. To make things more manageable, I usually pull out two to three goals at a time in different areas of my life and that may take different levels of commitment and time to focus on. The areas include: health, family, relationships, career, and life (fun stuff like getting a tattoo - which I haven't done yet!). Then, I look at the calendar and start setting a timeline and breaking down the steps I need to take. Some goals can be accomplished quickly (booking a ticket to Las Vegas), others can be multi-year projects like writing this book.

A famous study of Harvard graduates confirms that what I was doing intuitively - and what your nursing college is asking you to do by revisiting your goals on a yearly basis - is a key to goal success. The 1979 Harvard MBA class was asked "Have you set written goals and created a plan for their attainment?" The study concluded[6] that the 3% of the MBA graduating class who both wrote down their goals and had a plan made ten times more money as the other 97% put together, just ten years after graduation.

It's usually not enough to write down SMART, value-based, infinite-minded short and long-term goals if you shelve them, leaving the accomplishment to chance. You *have* to revisit that plan to stay the course or course correct as needed. The more connected your goals are to your values, the more vividly you describe your goals, and the more frequently you revisit your goals, the more likely you are to be successful.

EXERCISE: Planning for success

1. Look at the goals you originally set. Start with the goal that you feel either the most passionate about, you feel would make the biggest difference in your career, or the one that is easiest to achieve.
   - Under that goal write out the smaller steps you need to achieve it. Under those smaller steps determine if there are any micro steps you need to take.
   - Determine how much time you think each micro-step will take and the order in which they need to be completed. (Use a calendar, Gantt chart or list with dates for completion.)
2. Complete the following. I am on a mission to _____ and when I make this happen, I am going to celebrate by _____!!!
3. Make a plan to revisit your goals at least once a year. Block off the time in your calendar.

---

6 Lorsch, J. W., & Morse, J. J. (1985). Career paths and career success in the early career stages of male and female MBAs. Journal of Organizational Behavior, 6(4), 289-306.

You can go the conventional route and blend in. Or, you can stand out when you have the chance. You don't have to always play it safe.

MODULE 2

KEEPING YOUR CAREER INTERESTING

"Life is to be lived. If you have to support yourself, you had bloody well better find some way that is going to be interesting. And you don't do that by sitting around."

—Katharine Hepburn

By the end of Module 2 you will understand how to make your career interesting. Everything is interesting when it's new, but there are points in a career and nursing education that you may consider boring. This can lead to feeling unfulfilled and daydreaming about an exit from nursing. Disengagement, of course, also allows a greater possibility of making errors. After completing this module, you will be able to recognize boredom in your career, identify strategies for keeping your career interesting, and start putting the strategies to work for you.

RISKS OF A BORING CAREER

After the stress of my first year as a bedside nurse, I started to fantasize about spending the rest of my career in an office chair, working in an environment where my clients weren't all on the verge of death. I wanted my career to slowdown and be easier.

A "vanilla" career sounded like a dream: Commute. Clock in at 9 am. Do some work. Have a break. Relish in lunchroom gossip. Do some more work. Clock out at 5 pm. Get a pay cheque. Retire.

In search of a desk job, I applied to do data entry work in nursing research. "How well do you deal with boredom?" the interviewer asked. "Can you clarify your question?" I asked. "You've had an exciting career working in the emergency department and the intensive care unit - data entry is boring." Yes, ER and ICU, very exciting. But, didn't she know that boredom was the point? I *longed* for boredom! I wanted to tell her that I wanted nothing more than to spend all of my working hours in the warm glow of a spreadsheet that could not ask for a glass of water, demand a brief change, or require several rounds of CPR at a moment's notice. "I'm adaptable," I answered. The interview ended. I wasn't called back.

One year and several interviews later, I finally had the opportunity to work nine-to-five in the nursing leadership office of my hospital on secondment from my bedside role. My job was to cold call other hospitals, convince management to speak with me, and increase the uptake of completion of a research questionnaire on nursing staffing. Most of my calls were met with voicemail or annoyance. I dreaded picking up the phone. My fantasy was actually a bit of a nightmare.

I went from a high-risk, high-reward position to a low-risk, low-reward position.

While I was efficient at my work and I was successful in my role as far as the job description went, I wasn't passionate about it. After my tenure finished in the department, I wasn't offered any further opportunities and returned to the bedside with a new appreciation for my career.

We commonly hear about burnout in nursing however, we also need to recognize and prevent *boreout*!

Being under-stimulated at work may result in you feeling worthless. You become disengaged, depressed and anxious. The reality is that career boredom can be as devastating as burnout. Feeling bored should be considered a flashing "caution dead-end ahead" sign!

Nurses who are bored can either feel overworked or underemployed; both lead to distraction, tension, and disillusionment. Boredom also affects nurses' ability to focus and engage in their work leading them to no longer give their full attention or to run on autopilot. This can lead to costly and avoidable errors, bad patient outcomes, and low productivity.[7]

It may be no big deal to make an error like giving one, versus two, stool softener tablets but when you give one milliliter instead of one unit of insulin (100 times the dose) or give a full multidose vial of vaccine equivalent to six doses instead of drawing up just one dose, things get serious fast!

Thousands of patients die each year from medical errors. Health professionals are not perfect. If you've made an error, you're not alone and you've probably grown from the experience. If you haven't made a medical error, prevent it from happening by ensuring your career holds your interest and attention.

I can't tell you how many nurses I've met who are quietly counting down to retirement, whether it is 20 days or 20 years away! They've resigned themselves to fantasizing about the day they can hang up their scrubs. Despite having a lot of opinions on how to improve conditions

---

[7] Cleary, M., Sayers, J., Lopez, V. & Hungerford, C. (2016). Boredom in the Workplace: Reasons, Impact, and Solutions, *Issues in Mental Health Nursing*, 37:2, 83-89, DOI: 10.3109/01612840.2015.1084554

for patients and staff, these nurses avoid getting involved in efforts to improve working conditions, feeling that their efforts would be futile. You could see and hear their emptiness. Their career may not have started that way, but the work has become a means to an end.

Unfortunately, some of these same nurse colleagues have not made it to retirement. In a strange twist of fate, they wound up as a patient in the same hospital they worked in, never having a chance to relish retirement. Even though it was rare, seeing a former colleague in a hospital bed, providing them with their final bed bath, and transferring them into a white body bag to be taken to the morgue always hit home more than the other patients. It was even more depressing when I knew they were holding off on living their lives until retirement, meaning unrealized dreams.

Waiting until retirement to truly start living doesn't guarantee the ending you're hoping for. If you don't know how to enjoy life now, I promise you won't suddenly learn at age 65. And, if you aren't in good enough health to do all of the things you planned, like touring the Roman colosseum in Italy or strolling the Champs-Élysées in Paris by the time you hit retirement, that will be a shame. Enjoy the journey to retirement while you are still in good health. Take care of your mind, body, and spirit every day.

Having worked with some of the wealthiest people in Canada as an Executive Health Nurse Practitioner, I repeatedly heard that there is only so much golf you can play in retirement. Some individuals dabbled with retirement in their 30s and 40s after amassing enough wealth to support many future generations but, despite their financial wealth, many of these clients chose to return to work because they truly enjoyed what they did for a living.

You might be thinking, "What? Leave retirement? Did you check for a urinary tract infection because they must have been delirious!" Nope. You read that right! Their health and happiness were higher when working, than in retirement. That is what I want for you too. For you to make your career so interesting that you would consider never retiring.

EXERCISE: Boredom is no longer an excuse

1. Do your career pursuits interest you? Why or why not?
2. In your private life, identify the things that you like doing or used to like doing that give you energy and purpose.
   a. In what ways might you combine these interests with your career to create new, more exciting prospects for yourself?
3. If you haven't set your goals or they do not excite you, revisit the section on goal setting from Module 1.

CREATING INTEREST

Every emotion has a purpose. Once you've figured out that you're bored, your next job is to figure out the message.

Boredom feels negative and uncomfortable. We don't want to be bored, we want to be interested in, and excited about, what we are doing in our lives. The message of boredom is to redirect your attention to something new, different, and interesting.

When I think of boredom, I envision myself standing in thick mud. I don't want to stay in the mud. I want out! Hand me a shovel, I need to get to work.

In other words, take action and do something. Anything! Stop the boredom cycle by getting out of your head. Thinking about how bored you are, contributes to more boredom. You feel unmotivated. You stay stuck. So, break the cycle of negative thought, feeling, and inaction. Try:

- writing a list of things, you enjoy or want to try in the future.
- reading a book on a topic you want to learn more about; by another nurse author such as Tilda Shalof, or some brain candy you'd usually reserve for a tropical vacation.
- reaching out to someone you've lost touch with.
- sending a message on LinkedIn to someone whose career you admire, to open communication.

Consider talking about your feelings of boredom with a trusted colleague, mentor, career coach, or manager. Look for opportunities for education in an area of interest or to take on a new project. If there is nothing at your current job to keep you engaged, despite having these conversations, consider something on the side or leaving altogether. If you are promised a new project or title to keep you engaged but nothing changes in an agreed upon time frame, consider it a sign.

There is a misconception that you have to be miserable to quit your nursing job. You don't have to wait for burnout. You don't need to wait until you've taken your share of abuse. You don't need any justification. You get to quit because you decide to. Sometimes it's just time to move on because you want growth, new adventures or to try something else. That's ok! In fact, it's better than ok because you are not making a decision out of desperation.

Revisit your career goals. Do the career goals you set in the past still interest you? Have you stopped pursuing your goals? Did you achieve your goals and forget to set new ones? Identify a step you can take to move forward to achieving your goals or, with a new awareness of what you consider boring, come up with new goal. Let's get to work building that exciting career!

Now, a game of Q&A. I'm going to ask three questions. Write the answers here on the page, in a notebook or on the back of a grocery receipt.

1. What are you working toward right now?
2. What else are you working toward?
3. I think there is more. Give me one more thing you are working towards.

Thank you for playing! We've finished the game and you've identified three important things you're working toward right now!

Finding ways to make your life and career more of a game eases pressure. Time passes quickly when we're engaged in playing games and who doesn't love a little competition? "But Mary, nursing is serious business. It's not a game," you might be thinking. And, I agree. But what if you could reach the same positive outcomes with less stress and more fun?

Lighten up

When my husband and I started to think about names for our first son, I was very methodical. I looked at baby naming books, thought about initials, and considered the names of our grandparents. It was super stressful. There is so much weight in a name. After all, your name is with you for life!

"Thor," my husband suggested.

"As in the God of Thunder?" I replied.

"Yes," he said, very matter of fact.

With some reluctance, I agreed to name our son Thor. Now, I love introducing him to new people just to have the chance to say his name! I can promise you I would never have named my son Thor if it weren't for my husband. I would have tried really hard to fit in with Canadian naming norms. I would have *played it safe*. Thor would've been known as Michael "W" in a class full of Mikes or Jonathan "W" in a class full of boys named Jon. Instead, his name is strong, fun, and unforgettable!

The same applies to careers. You can go the conventional route and blend in. Or, you can stand out when you have the chance. You don't have to always play it safe.

Many people don't know this about me, but I had my lower lip pierced at age 15 and went through high school with multi-coloured or jet-black hair. I toned it down as I entered university and left my quirky side behind as I stepped into hospital clinical rotations. My program had a strict dress code and I complied. My identity shifted as I blended in, another nursing student in a sea of steel blue scrubs.

It wasn't until nearly ten years later when I relaxed the reins on my career and stopped worrying about the importance of titles like "ICU nurse" or "clinic director" that my career became more enjoyable. I started living "dangerously" by pursuing things that truly interested me and aligned with my values (like specializing in the area of medical cannabis).

Now, when asked what I have been up to, I respond, "I've been dabbling in...X." My career is a "choose-your-own adventure" game. My radar is always open to new career ideas and I will test the waters to see if they are right for me. I take joy in brainstorming new ways to help people and taking action to make it happen. Some side projects are successful, others are complete failures that I've been able to learn from. But, every once in a while, I strike gold! I discover something worth pursuing that I would not have found if I thought "career" meant only one job until retirement. Dabbling, being open and willing to try new things for better or worse, keeps my career fun and interesting.

Get passionate

Early in my career I didn't have any idea what I was interested in. I was in search of a "magical" something that would click and unlock career happiness. Nothing in nursing seemed to interest me. These days I call myself "multi-passionate" because I have *so many* interests. What changed? My perspective. Seeing infinite possibilities where I used to see limits.

You have to get excited to move the needle! As a Nurse Practitioner, one of my physician mentors was always excited about improving his patient's health, even if it was selling a curmudgeon of an old lady on the benefits of long-acting acetaminophen and fibre supplements. "Took your stool softener and had a soft stool, Mrs. Brown? Brilliant!" "Managed to get one extra hour of pain-free sleep? Wonderful!" His secret? He was passionate about healthy aging! He celebrated every small win that could lead to a better quality of life for his patients and had his patients do the same.

Some healthcare professionals give recommendations and hope for good outcomes, but this particular physician saw patient results as a worthy challenge and cracked the patient motivation code! I asked how he was able to get such positive results. He said, "Mary, anything short of a great result is a *disaster*!"

He was a little overzealous with his use of the word disaster, but it was evidence of a great passion for his work. He took the work of Steven Covey, author of *The 7 Habits of Highly Effective People*, to heart and was beginning the day with the end in mind! Every day he looked over his schedule and anticipated the challenges he would run into. He played out scenarios and full conversations in his mind to envision overcoming objections and putting the patient on the best route to success. Instead of dreading his full schedule, he embraced skipping lunch by calling it intermittent fasting and was excited to see how each imagined scenario played out in real life.

A lot of patients will nod in agreement when you give them a recommendation. They go home and return months—or even years later—with the exact same complaint, having followed *zero* of the recommendations. When you ask if they followed through, they will give you excuses. Time and money wasted.

If you, as a nurse, want someone to make a change—get them excited! Overcome their barriers and objections. We need to inspire sustainable change, achieved through motivation and measurable goals.

Let's use the example of that curmudgeonly patient with pain. Imagine they tell you they never started their treatment and can't understand why they still have pain. How do you feel when you hear this? Like, you're at square one or worse? Now, how do you think the patient feels? They may be nervous to talk to you knowing they didn't follow your advice. So, what can be done for them?

First, seek to understand, then you can seek to be understood. Become curious and ask why? On deeper questioning what if they reveal that they took their medication for a day and stopped because of constipation. The 5% relief in their pain didn't outweigh the drawback of constipation.

Now it's your turn. We better get it right this time or the patient is going to come back for a third visit without any progress or worse, not return at all.

First, celebrate any progress made. They took one dose and were willing to try, excellent! They got 5% relief, excellent! You can build on those small wins. Try to understand why they want the change and for whom? Ask what they don't like about the current state of their health and how it affects their closest friends or family. Then, have them participate in choosing the solution. Express empathy, help them to see that what they are doing now is not going to achieve the outcome they are hoping for.

Support their ability to change their lives. This brief motivational exercise not only works, it also gets results!

Now imagine *you* are the curmudgeonly patient and your major health concern is the state of your career. It won't be enough to say that you want to have your dream career. You can't go through the exercise of figuring out all the steps, only to leave your plan unrealized on paper. You deserve to have a career you are passionate about!

STOP AND THINK
How quickly can you move to the next step in your career? Picture yourself achieving your goals, and how you'll feel in your new life.

Small wins

In video games, as you advance the levels get harder. In life, the hardest part is often getting started. We all like to win so set yourself up for small successes. Get the serotonin boost. Then, the pressure will be off and you can move on to tackling more steps toward your goal. It's a long road and you have to get started.

When you are feeling stuck, it's likely not because you need a goal. If you've read this far and completed the exercises, you've established some goals. But, a big goal can be anxiety provoking.

Remember when you bought your first set of nursing textbooks? Each was as thick as your forearm. You wondered how you would ever get through just one, but you did! Each textbook was conquered page by page and lesson by lesson over the course of your studies.

When you are stuck, remember that you've been able to conquer big things before. Where possible set small goals that will start a momentum of success. Keep yourself in motion by minimizing stress and have fun along the way. I want you to experience win after win in the game of your nursing career. You're smart and capable!

EXERCISE: Gamify your career!

1. What can you do to make your career more like a game?
2. Apart from yourself, who are you building your career for? Who is playing the "game?"
3. List 20 things you are interested in. Now narrow that down to your top ten. Then, your top 3. Finally, your top 1. That is your passion!

OPPORTUNITY KNOCKS

TWENTY-ONE MONTHS—NEARLY TWO YEARS! THAT was the length of time my "opportunity radar" went into hibernation. My 2020 pandemic pregnancy and the first year of my eldest son's life took a toll on my professional motivation. I closed myself off to new opportunities and stopped writing this book which had been a nearly complete first draft.

Thankfully, as my son's first birthday approached, my motivation kicked back in. Getting some sleep took me from total zombie to returning from the dead. I started to think about returning to work. I knew I didn't want to return to my old job at the end of my 18-month maternity leave (thank you Canada for the great maternity leave laws). We were a year and a half into the pandemic. My gym business had been closed by the government for over 400 days and was nearing bankruptcy and I knew I wanted a full-time, permanent job where I could work from home.

I started paying attention to my usual channels for opportunities—online professional message boards, professional networking sites and online job postings that had been coming into my inbox since I set up notifications on the site. Within weeks an opportunity presented itself through my professional social network. I applied immediately and within a few days, had a full-time permanent work-from-home job offer for the same salary that I had been making in my in-person role.

What I want to make clear is I didn't *do* anything extra to find the opportunity. I didn't have to navigate online job postings daily or apply on a company website. From having built my career using the WISELY method, the wheels were always in motion whether I was paying attention or not. Once my attention shifted back toward awareness, the opportunity presented itself and it was up to me to take advantage of it.

Be open to opportunity

This book isn't just about finding the perfect job, it's about building a career full of opportunity! So, instead of *job* searching, we're going to talk about *opportunity* searching. Job searching is a narrow-focused and tedious process. The thought of it evokes visions of endless scrolling through help-wanted ads and facing endless rejection. On the other hand, opportunity searching is exciting, hopeful, promising, and actually quite fun! Repeat after me, "Opportunities come to me at regular intervals and I am open to them."

Have you noticed that just when you start to think about buying a snazzy new gold stethoscope you suddenly notice several nurses on your unit with one? This is the Baader-Meinhof effect or frequency bias.[8] When your awareness of something increases, you believe it is happening more. In reality, those gold stethoscopes were everywhere, you just didn't notice them.

The same applies to opportunities. When you become open to opportunities, you will start to spot them all around you, even though they have been there the whole time.

Opportunity searching involves keeping an open mind while looking for the next stepping stone toward your goals. Apart from the obvious job postings, an opportunity could also be: a course, a volunteer role, a seat at a board table, a conference to attend or present at, a podcast to be a guest on, or a business opportunity. Broaden your mind. Entertain ideas that seem unlikely, and look for opportunities to diversify.

For some opportunities, you will have to use traditional search methods like checking job boards, company job postings, and cold calling. Others, like the one that came up for me will come through the grapevine. The important point is that you have to be open to opportunities for you to notice them and take advantage.

---

8 Zwicky, A. M. (2006). *Why are we so illuded?* Retrieved January 28, 2023 from http://www-csli.stanford.edu/~zwicky/LSA07illude.abst.pdf.

Take action

When an opportunity presents itself and aligns with your goals and interests, don't delay. Apply! Inquire! Say yes - or at least maybe. Break through any resistance or fear that can otherwise keep you stuck. After all, resistance is just a little test from the universe to see how open to possibility you are. Persist through the hurdles meant to weed out less interested or motivated candidates. Pull the threads of the universe towards you by being first.

This advice applies to applications to school, volunteer organizations, for funding, or any other opportunity that is in alignment with your goals. Once you've made it a habit of communicating your interest, it becomes easier. Yes, your first application may be rejected, don't let that hold you back. Apply broadly as opportunities arise.

My husband gets annoyed whenever he offers me food and I say no. He knows if he asks a second time, I'm likely to say yes. It doesn't make sense to him why I wouldn't say yes in the first place. But this isn't a slice of cake knocking, this is your life. Don't wait for someone to ask twice. Think of job advertisements and calls for abstracts as invitations. You don't have to pretend you don't want a position and you don't have to act too proud or play coy. Be confident in your worth. If it's a course you're thinking of taking, don't delay. Once that class is full you might be waiting months for it to be offered again. In the case of cold calling prospective employers, you're not waiting for someone to ask, you're making the first move.

While I truly believe, *what is for you won't go past you*, I also believe that if you pass up an opportunity you may be waiting a long time for a similar opportunity to reemerge. Don't wait until you're 100% ready, 60-80% ready with a pull from your heart is good enough. I repeat, don't wait for someone to ask twice. You will gain a competitive advantage.

As an undergraduate, I was advised to apply for Registered Nurse positions in my final semester, months before I would have a license. I did and was rewarded with a job offer long before graduation. Then, as a Nurse Practitioner student, I was advised the same. Even though I didn't have my license and felt a bit silly applying for jobs I wasn't yet fully qualified for, I applied and again I was comfortably employed earlier than expected.

As difficult as it is, when it comes to career, your classmates will be your competition when looking for work. Employers hire people, not qualifications. If they like you and feel you fit the qualities they are looking for, they will wait for your credentials to come through. Psychologically, we remember people who go first. We give them slack if they aren't perfect, some credit for being brave, and we see them as ambitious. It's a natural competitive advantage.

Admittedly, I usually volunteer to go first because I am afraid rather than brave. I used to be someone who never raised my hand or asked questions. To have a successful career on my terms, those two qualities held me back. I am also an introvert by nature so sticking my head out is not my first inclination. Nonetheless, I have found my way by being first. No matter what your personality or how you were raised, you can be seen and heard by being first out of the gate.

It's natural to hesitate—it is your brain's safety mechanism to make sure you are making sound decisions. But don't get stuck. Failure to make a decision is still a decision. The consequences of passing up an opportunity out of fear can ripple through your life.

Rejection as opportunity

When you don't hear from an employer after submitting an application, do you consider the opportunity game over? If you have an interview and aren't hired, do you take it personally?

If you apply to a nursing program and don't get in on the first try, do you stop there? It's time to reframe those negative thoughts!

Don't be discouraged by rejection or silence. You never know when that application you submitted will bear fruit. Hiring cycles can be months long. I've been contacted *a year* after putting in an application.

As a hiring manager, I've reached out to applicants several months after their submission, when hiring freezes come on unexpectedly and then are later lifted. Some opportunities won't align with your ideal timing. Knock on all the doors and then keep those doors open. Continue to work on your personal and professional development rather than waiting.

If you receive a "no," ask what you can do to get into the program or win the position next time. Asking for feedback can be scary. When decision-makers see that you are serious about an opportunity, and willing to do the work before you get the "yes," they will understand your dedication to your goals or to their organization. This will only benefit you in the long run.

I promise the right opportunity will present itself when you are ready. What is for you won't slip away unless you let it.

EXERCISE: Take action

1. In the next week, identify three opportunities that may advance your career. (If you notice more than three opportunities, note if they have a similar theme.) If no opportunities suit you, drill down to the type of change you are seeking. Your subconscious will continue to look for you.

2. Create a customized cover letter and resume suitable for the opportunities you've found. If your resume needs updating, and you're unsure how best to proceed try an online search for examples or seek advice from a professional.

3. With each application ensure you have eliminated typos and have correct dates. Customize the "To" line to reflect the right company. Adjust skills and attributes to align with what the ad is looking for. Try to use their keywords as software is sometimes used to narrow down candidates. Submit your application according to the specifications of the job ad.

4. If there isn't a job available, submit a resume for consideration for future openings.

5. Follow up. Sometimes applications are lost or are at the bottom of a big pile. A professional follow-up can go a long way in having your resume make its way to the right set of eyes.

LATERAL MOVES

Nursing is unique. You can be a nurse, but work in thousands of different environments. You can hold the same title whether you care for babies, or the elderly, or for diabetic foot ulcers. You can tire of one area and move laterally to another area, and another, and another. You can make the same amount of money from shifts within your organization or, more money. (Such was the case of travel nursing during the COVID-19 pandemic. Travel nurses were often making 3-4 times more than their traditional employment positions.)

Lateral movement can be freeing or hold you hostage. It is freeing if you quickly need to find a new job or seek to keep your career interesting. At the same time, you can get too comfortable within your job band and repeated lateral moves may also make you an "unreliable" hire to employers.

As a novice nurse I waited for my annual sixty cent raise while making lateral moves within my department. I valued the experience, but after several years and specialization without additional compensation, my earning potential felt limited.

My friends outside of nursing were also making lateral movements. A friend in marketing went from start-up to start-up, negotiating higher salaries along the way. Inside of nursing, lateral moves in unionized environments such as the hospital where I started my career were rarely rewarded with more money. For example, I made the same amount of money as a medical-surgical nurse with no specialty training, as when I was an ICU nurse with additional critical care certification. Salary was based on years of experience and the collective bargaining agreement rather than an individual's level of specialized knowledge and expertise. All nurses under the agreement were valued the same. Generally, only when moving into leadership did one jump up the salary grid and there were no opportunities to break the ceiling of the grid for outstanding work.

Meanwhile, a friend in a non-unionized hospital had a different experience. She went from a general ward to an oncology ward and received a bump in pay, then a year later went on to ICU where she made several thousand more. Faced with the limitations of our respective organizations, we ultimately both left the public hospital system and moved into the private sector. Using her higher salary as a baseline, she easily negotiated her worth, while I struggled to understand what my value truly was. My mindset was fixed on the idea that the going rate was non-negotiable.

When considering moving into unknown waters in nursing, take the opportunity to negotiate enhanced pay and benefits. Whether unionized or not, be prepared to argue your worth and get compensated appropriately.

When making a lateral move—prepare as you would for your first interview, but your responses should reflect a deeper level of experience. It helps to keep track of significant stories of challenging clients and interpersonal relationships from your day-to-day work life. These stories may feel like they will be with you forever, but I promise you will forget them if you don't write them down.

STOP AND THINK

Write a reflection on your experience thus far, what you enjoy about your current work and what you long for in future opportunities.

Be prepared to answer questions about why you are seeking a shift from one environment or specialty to another. If you have limited experience in the area you are applying into, be prepared to discuss past experiences and your plan for moving forward. Show your value and initiative. You wouldn't be making a lateral move if you weren't motivated to do so. Make sure your interviewer is left with the impression that you are excited and a more worthy hire than someone who already has experience in the area you're looking to pursue.

Negotiation strategy

While working as a Nurse Practitioner, I was happily employed on a contract for maternity leave coverage. I knew the contract would be up in six months and was aware of the competitive market for Nurse Practitioner positions, so I kept my eyes open for job opportunities. One of the best ways I've found jobs over the years has not been from job search websites or company websites, but from word of mouth.

As luck would have it—luck being preparation meets opportunity—an opportunity was posted on an online message board by another Nurse Practitioner who I had met in the past. I reached out and learned about the position which was for a contract full-time role in my area of expertise. I told her I was looking for a permanent full-time role and she thought there may be an opportunity to negotiate what I was looking for. She gave me information about the company's background, what the position expectations were and why she felt the previous Nurse Practitioner left the position. She was gracious enough to outline the pay structure, and when I asked what she felt a reasonable request for salary might be, she recommended a number 20-25% below what I was making at the time. I told her I was still interested, because I don't like to pass up opportunities and she forwarded my curriculum vitae to the hiring manager.

A few days later I received an email from the Chief Operating Officer of the company to schedule an interview. (Do not get scared of titles, C-level executives are people too.) The email was clearly a copy-and-paste standard message that he sent in haste, neglecting to personalize or add a subject line. It read:

Hello Mary,

Thank you for your application on Indeed. We were impressed with your resume and would like to ask you some further questions to get to know you better.

> *First off, are you still interested in this position?*
> *Why are you interested in this role?*
> *When are you available to start?*
> *When is the best time to reach you for a phone interview?*
> *Are you open to a 12-month contract?*
> *What are your salary expectations?*
> *Do you have any vacations planned in the near future?*
> *Thank you, and I look forward to hearing from you soon.*
> *Regards,*

The errors and brevity did not stop me from replying professionally to each and every one of these questions, including the expected salary. I assumed the writer had good intentions but was busy or distracted at the time they sent the email. Always assume the positive and not the negative, giving your contact the benefit of the doubt. Here was my response:

> *Good morning,*
>
> *Thank you for considering me for the position of Nurse Practitioner.*
>
> *After hearing about the position, I am interested in interviewing and learning more about the vision for the future of the company.*
>
> *Having worked in the field since 2019, I find it very rewarding. My patients have seen tremendous success with managing the symptoms of their chronic conditions. Many patients return on follow-up with words of appreciation and tears of joy that their long-term issues are vastly improved.*
>
> *At this point in my career, I am looking for a full-time, permanent role with a salary of $xxx,xxx a year.*
>
> *I am available to start part-time within the next 2 weeks, moving to full-time after notice to my current employer is completed.*
>
> *I have a short vacation planned for the last week of August.*

I am available for an interview evenings after 7pm, anytime over the weekend, or June 28 or 29 between 9am-12pm. I can be reached by e-mail or text/phone at xxx-xxx-xxxx.

Looking forward to hearing back from you.

Sincerely,

Mary Ghazarian NP-PHC

If you are like me, you focus on the salary. I chose a salary number that was slightly aspirational. It was above my pay from the other company, but not offensive. If I had asked for the lower salary suggested to me, there would be no room for negotiation. I felt this number was justifiable as I knew contracting out this position would add an extra 20%. Also, I knew it left room for the employer to counter-offer and for us to hopefully meet somewhere in the middle.

In the end, I was offered the position, but not with enough salary or benefits to entice me from my current position. Instead, I used the offer to renegotiate with the company where I was already employed.

When making a lateral move, unless there are significant benefits, the goal should be to end up with a higher or equal salary rather than a pay cut. You want to be in a better situation than where you began. Do not start a negotiation low. Start high enough as to not offend the potential employer and not be disappointed with the outcome. The last thing you want is to have to look for another position again, because you failed to ask for what you needed. Employers and HR departments expect negotiation. They expect the salary you ask for to be higher than what will be agreed upon.

Lateral movement keeps your career interesting and can grow your earning potential quickly. Use lateral movement as a tool as you build your career.

EXERCISE: Planning a move

1. What would it take for you to leave your current position for a similar position in another area of practice or organization?

2. What is the minimum salary you would be willing to accept when making a lateral move? If that is your goal, where would you start your negotiation?

HOW *NOT* TO KEEP THINGS INTERESTING

I WENT TO WORK HUNGOVER ONCE and it was one time too many. It was the morning after a work holiday party, I had one or two glasses of champagne too many and was working on just a few hours of sleep. I spent the day feeling like I should be the patient in the bed. As luck would have it, I was assigned one of the most unstable patients in the unit. I could barely keep the patient's story straight for all of the specialists coming through. I vowed, "Never again!"

Every superhero knows, "with great power comes great responsibility." You may be trying to *keep things interesting* in your career by self-sabotaging or participating in some other unhealthy relationship with your work.

There are several types of career self-sabotage that give our brains a serotonin boost, but don't help in the long run. Some of these include: being a workaholic, disorganization, indecisiveness, perfectionism, procrastination, and having imposter syndrome. Some nurses also turn to substance abuse, attending work drunk or high to cope. These are not the type of ideas I have in mind when I advise to keep your career interesting.

Do you have that one friend who seems to get into the perfect relationship and then a month later is single again? They gush about their new lover, planning the engagement and saying they'll invite you to the wedding. Then, the next time you get together, they tell you, "It's over." They always seem to want to move too fast or too slow for their partner. Or, they got bored of their partner. Or, they reveal their partner cheated, just like their last three partners. What gives?

When you have an underlying paradigm that attracts you to opportunities that are not in your best interests, you end up in a negative pattern of making the same decisions that get you the same outcomes.

If you are hopping from one job to another and not finding "the one," or are stuck in the same job you have been complaining about for years, you have to examine the reason why this is happening. Is it boredom?

Feeling overworked? Feeling underpaid? Do you have an abusive manager? Is it perfect, but you don't feel you deserve an opportunity in line with your ambitions so you subconsciously mess it up and get fired? If you want a different outcome, you need to identify the cause and you have to interrupt the loop.

Career self-sabotage is an abusive pattern toward yourself. You actively or passively block the achievement of your career goals.

I first learned about the intimate partner cycle of violence as a nursing student working in a women's shelter. In an emotionally or physically abusive relationship, there is the honeymoon phase, a tension-building phase, a crisis phase, and then a honeymoon phase again as the cycle repeats.[9] People experiencing intimate partner violence will attempt to leave several times before they are finally successful.

Similarly, it may take multiple attempts to leave a job where you are feeling disengaged, burnt out, underappreciated, or abused. Most jobs start out in the honeymoon phase. You are excited to take on a new challenge and are offered support during your orientation. However, some managers or employers will try to get everything they can out of you. You know you may be better off elsewhere, but stay for the pay cheque and security. Your boss may convince you things will change. They promise a raise, increased staffing, newer supplies, or free education. But, if those promises aren't delivered, or don't move the needle for you, you need to leave.

Ensure that you don't finally leave your job only to jump into another position with similar pitfalls. That would be self-sabotage. Do your research. Determine what has gone wrong for you in the past. Before taking on a new role, speak with others doing similar work in the organization where you are hoping to be hired.

---

9 Vetter, C., Devore, E. E., Wegrzyn, L. R., Massa, J., Speizer, F. E., Kawachi, I., Rosner, B., & Walker, L.E. (1984). *The Battered Woman Syndrome*. New York, Springer Publishing Company.

What if your employer or manager is excellent? They pay you fairly. They deliver on promises. They keep the unit well-staffed. They even pay for lunch once a week—a real unicorn of a job. Too good to be true? Your brain may think so and again, self-sabotage may rear its ugly head.

What if you're self-employed or you're a student? You are your own boss. There is no one to treat you good or bad but yourself, yet this is the most common self-sabotage relationship. There is no physical third party involved, only the voice in your head.

When you are bored, your brain may ask you to test the barriers. You may get a serotonin rush from arriving late for work or procrastinating on completing an important project to see if you can just skate by. You may seek substances to dull negative emotions or enhance positive ones. These are dangerous to you personally and professionally.

Ultimately, recognizing that *you* are in control of your destiny can start you on the path to leaving a cycle of disorganization, indecisiveness, perfectionism, procrastination, imposter syndrome, or any other self-sabotage you can identify.

We'll dive deeper into changing mindset in future modules. If you are having issues with substance abuse, contact your local crisis line for resources.

STOP AND THINK

Is there anything you are doing in your career that is not in your best interest? Have you ever self-sabotaged your nursing career or education?

"Nursing more and doing less" is accomplished by setting up systems to help the most people possible without needing to be physically present 24/7.

MODULE 3

SUSTAINING A SUCCESSFUL CAREER

"Begin with the end in mind."
—Steven Covey

By the end of this module, you'll have the tools to craft a sustainable career while thinking about the legacy you want to create for others. For many, sustainability is an afterthought that only comes at either a crisis point, or retirement. Planned sustainability is something you can work towards throughout your career, helping to smooth transition points while providing a compass for important decisions.

WHAT IS SUSTAINABILITY?

HAVE YOU BEEN RUNNING YOURSELF into the ground to accomplish your goals or to meet the needs of everyone around you? Not taking time for yourself to recharge, let alone empty your bladder? How long do you think you can continue until you burn out altogether?

Many self-help books are full of advice on how to do more and sleep less, but sleep deprivation is a form of torture that I can't get on board with! Other books include images of beach vacation photos and offer the opposite advice of "do less, get more" as if your dreams will all come true once you can learn to just chill out. What am I proposing instead? Plan for sustainability.

Your career is a marathon, not a sprint. This means finding ways to sustain yourself long-term in all facets of your life: professional and personal, relationships with organizations and your community, and financial considerations.

I first learned about sustainability during week 11 of a 12-week fellowship in project management. Too little too late! At the time, I had just completed my project, a nursing conference. After charging only $20 a head, there was no profit to reinvest into a future event—not a sustainable pricing strategy. If there was one thing I could go back and redo, it would be to factor into a budget how much would be needed to repeat the conference the following year. I could've set the price higher and secured sponsors but money intimidated me and *my* low self-worth was reflected in the registration fee. We'll get to money blocks in Module 5.

Luckily, sustainability took care of itself. The conference built a sense of togetherness and belonging to the Nursing Resource Team nurses who otherwise felt they had no home base. While I had done the work to make it happen, the success of the conference had been all theirs. The attendees had embraced the experience, making it bigger than I had envisioned it ever could be. At the end of day two of the conference, I was approached by nursing leadership from other hospitals asking to host the event the following year. Three volunteering organizations took over the organization of the event in subsequent years.

The next year, I helped build capacity by consulting from a distance. I let go of the reins and saw my project soar. I was happy as a bedside nurse attendee, instead of a host or speaker, witnessing the energy in the room from another vantage point. I attended a third year with a poster presentation in hand. I left the NRT after that and trusted the conference would proceed without me as I moved on in my career. I don't know if the conference ever became profitable. But, for a short while at least, I knew it was sustainable.

After traditional retirement, Claudia Mariano former head of the Nurse Practitioners Association of Ontario continued to stay connected with the next generation NPs. She was pulled back to mentor and in the process created new opportunities for herself as a consultant. Sustainability in retirement usually refers to having enough money to live comfortably. I would argue that retiring with enough interest in the profession to continue to stay involved, is the sign of a successfully sustainable career.

Sustainability has many meanings; that you as an individual will continue to see a project through, or profitability. It also can mean continuing to bring value into the future, or creating an enduring legacy.

EXERCISE: Consider sustainability in your career

1. What brings you joy?
2. Is there any one thing you keep coming back to, or has been on your "wishing to accomplish" list?
3. What do you know to be true that you are not yet pursuing with full conviction?
4. What will be the thing that will make your career sustainable?

TIME FREEDOM

WORKING HARD IS NOT A problem. Nurses are basically married to hard work. It is not your work ethic that you need to sharpen, but the *direction* of your effort and your success habits.

- Are you doing the right things to get the outcomes you are looking for?
- Are you following the agenda of others or your own?
- Are you wasting time scrolling through your junk mail instead of checking something off on your success to-do list?

I'm often asked how I manage to do so much. The answer is not what you may think. This book was not completed with 8-hour days at a computer in a secluded log cabin overlooking snow-capped mountains as I often fantasized about. Instead, it came together in focused 15-minute periods between the responsibilities of being a business owner, nurse practitioner, partner and mother.

Before motherhood, I wasn't a great manager of my time. Tasks often took up as much time as I could give them and I would procrastinate, barely meeting deadlines. Managing time takes a good planner and I was more of a *pantser*—I flew by the seat of my pants. Motherhood showed me being a pantser could only get me so far. Things had to change if I was going to handle both motherhood and a career.

We all have responsibilities to juggle. Pre-motherhood, my plate was already full. I was working 60+ hours a week, plus had a 1–2-hour daily commute. I went to the gym two evenings a week. This left me with very little time for everyday life stuff, like grocery shopping, meal prep, and a third or fourth weekly workout I desperately wanted. Time with my husband, friends, and family fell by the wayside. I made a lot of money, but I also *wasted* a lot of money to make up for my lack of time. "If I only had more time," I thought.

I looked forward to maternity leave as I thought it would allow me to focus and grow some of the creative ideas that had been circling in my mind and scribbled in my notebooks. As luck would have it, life had other plans. The pandemic struck.

Due to pandemic restrictions for gyms and grossly inadequate government support for small businesses, my two income-earning fitness studios became money-eating machines. My maternity leave funds would not be sufficient, so I returned to work three months after the birth of my son. Between working 40 hours a week, breastfeeding every 2-3 hours day and night, preparing meals, cleaning, and finding time for my husband, there was very little time left for myself, my career pursuits (like writing this book), or taking on private clients for health or career coaching. I could no longer do it all myself.

I hired a nanny I couldn't afford and enlisted grandma to help. I quietly mourned the loss of a normal pregnancy and postpartum period and shelved the partially finished manuscript of this book. I had to reprioritize time, money, and energy.

When I became a mother, the number of hours I could dedicate toward my career goals drastically reduced, but my career goals didn't change. I had lost the income from the gym and my part-time job but knew that I could never go back to working the many extra hours now that I was a mother. If I wanted to earn the same income as pre-motherhood, I would have to find another way. I couldn't steal those hours from my family. As the wisdom goes—no one lies on their deathbed wishing they had spent more hours at work.

Approaching my son's first birthday, I was finally getting sleep and regained the desire to finish this book but still didn't know where to find the time. Before motherhood, I imagined I could pull a J. K. Rowling and write in the mornings before my son woke up, but I was stuck with a 5 am earlier riser—like mother, like son—so getting time for myself in the morning was out of the question. Instead, the only child-free time I had was 7-10 pm, 5 nights a week (since I worked evenings the other two).

My husband and I were in the habit of spending evenings on the couch watching brain candy reality tv shows but instead of feeling relaxed and connected to my husband as I had pre-baby, I would feel anxious. I felt there were other things I needed to be doing for myself and our family—things like writing and creating another income stream. I felt guilty for not being able to enjoy my husband's company during the little time we had to ourselves. Truth be told, sometimes he would guilt me about it too. We both felt the squeeze of my schedule, new parenthood, and the pandemic. I was frustrated but nervous to tell my husband about my needs but with no other solution, found a quiet moment and started with the dreaded, "Honey, we need to talk." I explained I would be cutting TV time down from three hours to one hour. I explained my goal of completing my book and told him how it would benefit him.

"The book would be like a mini clone of myself," I said. I would have more freedom. With a product like a book or online course, you finish the work once and then it goes out into the world, earning money and opening doors. After having children, I didn't have time to coach as many nurses or see as many patients, but I still had the desire to impact more lives. Publishing the book would be a time, money, and opportunity multiplier.

To my surprise, he was in agreement. He had noticed how stressed I was and hadn't wanted to be the one to bring it up. He appreciated my honesty and sharing my needs instead of letting the issue fester. He could see the short-term sacrifice would ultimately lead to more time for our family.

80/20

Instead of spending 100% of your time in clinical nursing, (or whatever your main job duties are) what if you could spend 80% of your time on your main job duties and 20% of your time on quality improvement, education, or other projects that interested you? And I'm aware that many of you may be spending not just 100%, but 120% of your time on your main job duties! You are *overworking* in aspects of your career that move the needle forward for your patients and the organizations you work for, but not for your long-term professional growth.

So how do we get from 120% down to 80/20? It begins by taking control of the 20%. Reserve time for actions that get you closer to your goals. Block it off and dedicate the time *before* you even think you have it available. At first, this may require using your personal time. But as you recognize the benefits of this approach, you will look for ways to make this sustainable by: speaking with your manager about incorporating education hours and quality improvement hours into your job duties, talking to the chief nursing officer about creating an organization-wide 80/20 project for nurses, or building a nursing business that allows you to make up for lost income if you cut your main work hours to part-time.

Time management

For my 15th birthday I received a black, hard-cover day planner better suited to someone much older. However, in my abundant spare time as a teenager, I pulled out the planner and started to plot out my days: 6 am-wake up, 7 am-catch the bus. I added each of my high school courses and their respective time slots, my part-time job, studying, school projects, assignments, and reading. I used a different highlighter for each activity. Finally, I had a full technicolor schedule. I could see the blank spaces representing my free time and planned for those too— so no space would be left blank. I repeated the exercise every week until the pages ran out, then I bought a new one.

I stopped using day planners after I finished my Bachelor's degree, but periodically I get back to basics when I feel stressed. If I don't have a fancy day planner, I take out a blank piece of paper and draw a grid with the days of the week across the top and hours down the side. I colour block the time I have. These days, time is allocated for my family, my day job, chores, paying bills, and sleep. As I gaze at my masterpiece, a crucial category is often missing. Myself!

We need to stop saying, "I need more time" and instead become aware of how we spend our time. Then we can get intentional with our choices—focusing on structuring the time that we available.

At a certain point, there are no more hours to trade for money, especially for work you don't enjoy. Time spent writing makes me happy. I get into a flow state and time flies. My stress decreases and I feel filled with purpose but I know that I can't spend all my time writing for fun or again, there is no time for anything else. Sustainability is about balance. Sometimes work will take priority, sometimes life. Accepting the ebb and flow. Planning for a brighter future will make your career more sustainable.

Delegation

As a bedside nurse, I was guilty of doing *all* the jobs. I avoided calling the care assistant to help me turn a patient because I didn't want to add to their workload. I emptied the garbage bins instead of calling housekeeping. I answered phones when they could have been left to the secretary. Seems innocent, right? Not so. I was scared to delegate and naive to the consequences of doing these tasks myself. I could have hurt myself turning a patient alone. I could've been reprimanded for emptying garbage cans in a unionized environment, as I was technically robbing my colleagues of work. By the end of the day, I was rushed to chart and was forced to stay late.

Stop doing *all* the things. It's not sustainable. Start delegating. Own your expertise and pass on the rest to those who can do it more efficiently and for fewer dollars an hour than you. Reserve your talents for the things that really need to be done *by you*. I'm not advocating dumping all of your tasks on others. I'm encouraging you to empower others by giving them the opportunity to be productive. Manage your workload so you can function optimally.

Don't get me wrong, you still need to lead by example and be a team player. Do tasks outside of your area of expertise from time-to-time to stay grounded and aware of what you are asking of others—not to take over their roles. Delegating helps to grow confidence and immediately increases progress. You don't need to work alone. Build up those around you and accept support.

Nurse more, do less

Nurses are taught that our value has a lot to do with our physical presence at the bedside. You might have entered this profession thinking, "I want to help everybody." Unfortunately, you *can't* help everybody. The world census just passed 8 billion. Even if you spent all 24 hours being physically present with as many people as possible, you would still not be helping them all. You have to accept the limitations of traditional nursing roles. All of your day can't be spent directly with clients. Time needs to be spent on education, documentation, planning, teaching, learning, and tending to your own biological needs.

If you're working at the bedside, plot out your 12-hour shift and see how you're spending your time. Are you making unnecessary trips to the supply room? Getting paged by patients for ice chips all day long? Could you set up a system with your colleagues that is more efficient?

If you're in an office working 8-hour days the same applies. Are you spending unnecessary time on social media? Are you involved in any redundant meetings? Could you accomplish the same or more working from home? Can you negotiate the number of days you commute into the office? Are there tech tools that could streamline your tasks? How are you spending your break?

"Nursing more and doing less" is accomplished by setting up systems to help the most people possible without needing to be physically present 24/7.

I think back to nights shifts where I spent wasted hours browsing online for nicer apartments and the perfect all-inclusive vacation—just trying to stay awake. Those quiet hours (I know, never say the "q" word in a hospital) would have been better spent doing something more productive such as creating resources for patients or colleagues. But, the concepts of sustainability and income beyond my hourly rate weren't in my awareness.

To earn more money and serve more people in a day, you will need to do the work to build the system, write the book, create the online course, invest your money, or train employees to do what you do. You will need to eke out extra time in your day to build your foundation. But, once accomplished, your time will be free for other pursuits. It's time to plan for a future where you can serve more people in your 24 hours.

EXERCISE: Find the time to do the thing

1. What are you doing now that can be delegated so that you can work in your zone of genius?
    a. Who can you delegate to?
    b. What are the costs of delegating?
    c. What are the costs if you don't delegate?
2. Write out your week with the days of the week across the top and hours in the day along the side. Fill in your schedule for each day of the week.
    a. Are you spending your time the way you would like to be spending it?
    b. Are there enough hours in the day for the things that matter most to you?
3. How can you free up time now, and in the future?
4. How can you multiply yourself?

CREATING CONNECTIONS: SUPPORT, FELLOWSHIP, AND NETWORKING

IF YOU ARE AN INTROVERT like me, you may find it challenging to initiate conversation or maintain more than a few close relationships. You may find it easier to hold entire detailed conversations with the voice in your head. Extroverts, you likely have no idea what I'm talking about! Regardless of your social inclination, connections with others are pivotal to your nursing career.

Support and fellowship

If you want to know what nurses really want out of their lives, speak with them on the night shift. In the wee hours of the morning, nurses become great philosophers. We find ourselves talking about moving the needle in health care, futile care, ideal staffing ratios, better compensation, and so on. The conversations are cathartic and serve to bond the night shift nurses together. Once in a while, however, an idea is born that gets to see the light of day.

After a 2am lament about the challenges I faced as a nurse floating through the hospital, I found that my colleagues all agreed with me. Rather than leave well enough alone, I brought the conversation to the round table of the unit council. The nurse educator recommended I make a plan to find solutions. I made a proposal for a workshop project that gained the support of the hospital. One hundred nurses and nurse leaders from across southern Ontario gathered for "Successes, Strengths, and Solutions," a day of sharing stories that may have otherwise been left on the night shift.

This was the first project beyond the bedside, that I worked on. After a detailed application for a quality improvement project, eight lucky bedside nurses were selected for an "80/20" project that pulled us from the bedside to work on a project of our choosing, with the support of a project manager. Some nurses worked on research, others on education, and I built a conference. We had all experienced different journeys in our careers, but were in pursuit of something greater than ourselves. We were doing things we had never done before. To navigate the challenge, we met every week to check in and learn from each other.

The fellowship group's leader, Carolyn Plummer, introduced *The Art of Possibility: Transforming Professional and Personal Life* by Rosamund and Benjamin Zander. This was the first time I was exposed to a self-help book. It felt a little silly, but we all went along with the activities suggested in the book. We started by scoring ourselves "A+" for our projects before we had even started the work. We were all high achievers and there was no other possibility than success, if that was our aim. The mind shifts that occurred in that room had the power to push us forward to meet our goals.

We were all immersed in (and learning) project management for the first time. At the weekly check-ins, there were more tears than you would expect. We poured our souls into our work and supported each other through other life challenges including loss, wedding planning, and pregnancy. We shared energy to power through "one more week" toward the next item on our project schedules. Without this group support, none of the projects would have seen the light of day and would have remained ideas in the heads of bedside nurses. This begs the questions,

- Who are you spending your time with?
- Are they aware of your goals and dreams?
- Are they supportive?
- Are they also pursuing their goals and dreams?
- Do you motivate each other and hold each other accountable? Or, are you holding each other back?

The group of peers you had in the past who got you to where you are today, may not be the peers you need to get where you are destined to go. Is there anyone you need to add? Anyone you need to let go of?

You cannot control anyone else, but you *can* control who you let into your circle. The people in your circle will directly influence how your brain works, and what you give attention to. If you have a circle focused on gossip instead of on big ideas, you are not spending mental energy focusing on the steps that could be moving you toward your dream goal.

Include a mentor in your circle, whether formal or informal. You should have someone you can consult, or confide in, who is a step ahead of where you want to be—not necessarily so that you can follow in their footsteps, but so that they can help *your* path unfold.

Build a circle that will propel you toward your goals, filled with people who won't judge you for tears, and who will help you get clear on your direction so that you can keep moving forward toward your vision for career success.

Networking

I have attracted many aligned opportunities through my network.

Before I published a book or had work accomplishments to be known for, I heard my name coming up through the grapevine on a semi-regular basis. "Do you know Nadine? We used to go to elementary school together. She says hi," or "Do you know Duane? He says you're pretty well known for your nursing advice."

Your network starts to organically grow when you are a nursing student. Over time, your network will be made up of colleagues, employers, and mentors. My network grew more formally as I invested time into growing my network online. Reaching out to nurses I admired and offering support to those who were looking for advice. At some point, the balance switched from those I met on the job, to being mostly made up of nurses I had never even met in person. Unlike the relationships in my inner circle, I may not communicate with members of my network on a regular basis, only connecting through social media but each connection has the potential for opportunity.

Healthcare is a small world that includes nurses, physicians, physiotherapists, respiratory therapists, naturopaths, chiropractors and more. In the long term, it is best to keep on good terms with as many as possible because you don't know what doors they could open or close for you.

In what way do you want people to talk about you? Positively or negatively? Your formal and informal network can be a blessing or a curse depending on how others perceive you. Being aware of this can help you to shift the narrative toward the positive and open doors in your career. For example, many jobs aren't posted because they are filled through word of mouth. Even if an opportunity *is* formally posted, I have found more success when someone in my network brings it to my attention because they are bringing me an opportunity they feel is aligned with my talents or interests. And, a strong, personal reference to the hiring team can go a long way toward floating you up in a sea of applicants.

When it comes to networking, work with your strengths. I'm an introvert, but I love connecting with people. I am not a natural face-to-face networker. For all of my expertise and despite a desire to improve, I'm really quite terrible at small talk. Following a lecture at a conference, I am not the type of person to walk up to the speaker for additional questions or to let them know I admire their work. I need time to reflect and digest information before building the confidence to come forward. I also have difficulty hearing in crowds. I am much more comfortable networking one-on-one over a drink or in writing by e-mail or direct message. So, I reserve my collegial energies for these types of interactions.

Online groups through professional associations or on social media platforms can connect you with other like-minded nurses. You can learn from nurses who are in the type of roles you are seeking or who are even in a position to hire. On social media, hierarchy is lost and leaders who participate in social media become accessible. In fact, I've had the pleasure of having nurses with great national and international experience reach out to me after seeing my work online. The great thing about social media is you never know who is watching. So, used wisely, it is a great networking tool.

Networking through volunteer work is another way to open doors. Attend professional association interest groups, volunteer to assist at nursing conferences or serve on special projects calling for nursing opinions and expertise. Take the opportunity to meet other like-minded, ambitious nurses and nurse leaders. These activities also add to your resume, which you should be growing even as a student or when unemployed.

Networking works best when you don't just take, but have something to offer. As a novice, you can start by letting people know you admire what they are doing. Comment positively on their opinions and indicate that you'd like to help in any way you can. As you develop expertise, you can contribute in a more substantial way. Think of what you can offer, even if it is simply to connect others.

Networking isn't just about building new connections, but also nurturing old ones. I once had a client tell me that the worst thing in life was to become irrelevant. When he retired, he lost touch with his entire network. He felt incredibly lonely and purposeless. Keep yourself visible and top of mind for others by connecting on a regular basis. Rekindle old relationships in a meaningful way. For example, one of the first things I did as a new grad NP was to keep in touch with a network of NPs on an online message board. I started meaningful conversations about independent practice and answered questions from other message board members based on my knowledge and experience. That group that I moderate has grown to over 1000 NPs.

Whether you consider yourself an introvert, an extrovert, or somewhere in between, connecting to others in your own authentic way is key to a sustainable career in nursing. Reflect on your current inner circle and bigger network. Make time to thank the people who have supported you. Complete the following exercise to get a better understanding of your current social circle and strategize how to grow it to support your goals.

EXERCISE: Your network

1. Who is in your inner circle?
2. Are the people you spend the most time with positive influences in your life?
3. Do you have a close circle of peers who boost each other up, move each other forward toward their goals and celebrate wins together? If not, how could you create one?
4. Are you introverted, extroverted, or a combination of the two?
5. How do you find it easiest to meet people?
6. List five ways you can build your network offline and online. Include how you can reconnect with old colleagues or mentors.
7. What can you offer to your network?

FINANCIAL SUSTAINABILITY

PRIOR TO THE EVENTS OF 2020, I was burning the candle at both ends with a full-time, traditional role in a medical office and a part-time job working from home throughout my pregnancy. "Will you quit your part-time job this week?" asked my husband. Every week I said, "Just give me one more week."

Despite the very real possibility of burning out yet again, I loved my part-time job in medical cannabis and fully intended to stick it out to make it my full-time gig when the opportunity arose. After COVID-19, our saving grace was my online gig!

While medical clinics pulled back hours and scrambled to pivot to virtual consultations, the medical cannabis company I was working for was already set-up for virtual work. Needs increased in medical cannabis, as people began avoiding medical clinics and emergency departments.

The pandemic brought out the worst and best in healthcare. Holes in healthcare systems the world over were exposed. Despite shortages of the nursing workforce in sectors like long-term care, cuts to nursing salaries and jobs were made. Some nurses dug deep and leaned into their resilience skills. Many others left the profession with varying degrees of disillusionment - some within three months of starting their first jobs.

With so much uncertainty at the best of times, how can you sustain your career even in the worst of times?

1. Embrace technology.
2. Have multiple income streams.
3. Be ready to pivot.
4. Have financial goals.

Embrace technology

If Florence Nightingale returned to earth, she would not recognize today's nursing profession. With the exceptions of continued emphasis on hygiene and a renewed focus on air purification; the landscape for nursing has changed dramatically. Electronic medical records, IV pumps, smart technology, remote monitoring, telecommunications and the internet have all disrupted traditional practice. With artificial intelligence and virtual reality starting to take off, the future possibilities to combine nursing and technology are endless.

The adoption of new technology follows a bell curve. There are the innovators, early adopters, early majority, late majority, and the laggards. Most people fall somewhere in the middle. To take advantage of new opportunities, you want to be a part of the beginning of the adoption curve, not late to the game.

Keeping up to date with how to use new technology and joining innovative healthcare companies can be daunting and uncertain. Not all technology sticks around, and not all companies do either, but the experience can be invaluable and every once in a while, a tech start-up takes off.

Nurses are not just users of technology, but also creators. The intersection of nursing and technology offers great opportunities to innovate. Connect with companies who are building the future of global health and offer your unique nursing perspective or investment dollars. Nurses are deeply connected with the needs of individuals, communities and societies which makes them ideal consultants and investors.

Create multiple income streams

It's hard enough to manage one full-time nursing position. Why am I asking you to take on two?

Well, I'm not. Income streams come in many forms. Traditional or self-employment inside or outside of nursing, contract work, product sales, affiliate sales, the stock market, and real estate investing are all examples of possible income streams.

If a lay-off comes your way before you're ready for retirement, what is your plan B? Are you planning to find another surgical nursing position? What if all elective surgeries are on hold as was the case during the pandemic? You will need to make money in another way.

It's not always the right season for building multiple income streams but when you have the motivation, take hold of it to pandemic-proof your career. If you haven't already, revisit your career goals and build in strategies for multiple income streams. Start to figure out what skills you need to build wealth and take the pressure off your full-time job. If you already are doing this, consider paying it forward by teaching other nurses what you know.

If you don't have the money to invest in something like the stock market or a mortgage, take advantage of low-cost or free options that only involve an investment in your time and energy. Build yourself a professional website, create content and make online courses. A few topics that you might be qualified to create content for: navigating the health system, controlling diabetes with lifestyle, navigating new parenthood, or how to build wealth for nurses.

Be ready to pivot

Pivoting is when you change direction in a significant way. The key to being able to pivot is being open to possibility, and recognizing that change is inevitable. Take advantage of new opportunities and abandon what isn't working.

When the pandemic hit and our gyms were forced to close, my husband and I didn't sit and twiddle our thumbs. We moved our business online offering virtual personal training sessions. We nurtured our client base so they would come back when we were able to reopen, and we paid our staff the best we could to ensure they were taken care of. We went from earning tens of thousands a month to just a few thousand, and government support was non-existent. With constant promises of reopening, we initially took out business loans to cover costs but a year later —with gyms still closed— we found ourselves at the end of our funds.

Rather than be forced to close, we got creative and used the last of our funds to hire a lawyer to find a way to reopen. We learned that the only population allowed to access gyms were persons with disabilities. With the blessing of the lawyer, we advised our staff of the changes and started advertising to individuals living with a disability requiring physical therapy by prescription. Within thirty days of considering calling it quits, our gym was full and we were on our way to repaying our loans.

During the pandemic, we weren't the only savvy business owners in my network. When Weighted-for-You custom weighted blankets orders dried up, the company—led by a former personal support worker—pivoted to making custom fabric facemasks. Fabric was in short supply due to shipping delays, so they had an advantage with their large stock. Instead of staying in their lane, they started to fulfill a new need in the market and earned twice as much as they had in the previous year.

Financial goals

How many overtime shifts equals one trip to Cabo?

Did you need to make the calculation or did you already know that number? How much time have you spent planning your next vacation compared to your financial future?

My husband lost both of his parents by the time he was 35. They passed away from cancer in their late fifties. So, for him, imagining a financial future that extended beyond the age of sixty was difficult. Having a child changed all of that. Now, he sees our financial future as *a legacy*.

It can be hard to imagine yourself living to the age of 95 and predicting the amount of money you would need to do so comfortably. Also, we know that anything can happen to cut your life short so what about living for the moment?

If you work with seniors, you understand what your future may hold and how much that depends on your financial situation. Staying in your home with the help of a private personal support worker may take more savings than moving into a publicly funded retirement home. Also, moving in with your children or grandchildren may or may not be an option. Many people are continuing to work beyond retirement because they either failed to plan, or extenuating circumstances changed the trajectory of their earning potential.

Speak with a financial planner to tease out the income you need—not just for an ordinary retirement, but for an *extraordinary* retirement. Then, strategize how to get there. This can mean leaner spending or increasing your earning potential, or both. Without an amount to aim for, you won't be able to understand the impact your present income will have on your future. The goal is to understand the numbers so you can set the bar. Then, as always, I want you to set it higher so that you can't miss.

Don't forget about inflation. Each year the cost-of-living increases, and the value of the dollar decreases. A dollar in your savings account from ten years ago has significantly less buying power today. When I went to the corner store as a five-year-old I could get 100 pieces of candy with a dollar. Today, the same candies are five cents each.

When it comes to financial sustainability, I want you to think beyond about what you need to live out the average life expectancy, instead, think of what you need to leave a financial legacy. It's true that you can't take money with you, at the same time, you don't want to run out of it either.

EXERCISE: Knowing the numbers

1. Write down your current sources of income.
   a. Where does it come from?
   b. How many hours of your time are required to produce that income?
2. Calculate the income level you will need to live comfortably beyond retirement; factoring in inflation, private home care, and other expenses that would make your life more comfortable.
3. Go a step further. Calculate what it might cost to live in Florida six months of the year because your arthritis will flare every winter in a cold climate, or add in the cost of a yacht and butler. Go big with your imagination and allow yourself to dream of outlandish possibilities. Feel what it would be like to have the financial means to support these dreams.
4. You may find a discrepancy between your income and what you need for even the most basic of retirements. Identify opportunities to increase your income in the following categories: employment, self-employment (creating your own income streams through entrepreneurship), and investing, as well as areas for saving.

LEGACY

Have you considered your legacy? It is a fairly loaded concept. Most of us will be forgotten within a few generations. Before I had clarity about what this meant in my life, legacy felt like a weight on my chest that I couldn't lift. Pondering legacy forced me to start thinking beyond retirement and to future generations.

If you've been following along, you know that I find future planning really exciting! When you allow yourself to imagine all of the possibilities and start to investigate how you can make them a reality, the weight lifts and your heart can start to flutter—metaphorically.

This step adds a layer to our goals that didn't exist before. We are going to talk about how to choose an area of practice where you can be of the greatest service *and* leave a legacy.

Legacy is what you leave behind and what you will pass down to others. As the founder of modern nursing, Florence Nightingale's legacy was her transformation of health care. As the project manager of your nursing career, you are in the privileged position to determine what will be left behind when you retire.

I sometimes wonder if the origins of the conference I founded were forgotten after the inaugural event, if my name ever surfaced in discussion or if it was lost in the bigger picture. Legacy was not something I thought about at the time, or even knew to think about. The conference was just the first proof that I could create something bigger than myself, bigger than impacting one life at a time, one nursing shift at a time. I learned that by positively impacting the nurses who are the backbone of understaffed, behemoth hospitals, ripples for the entire organization are created.

I choose to believe I left a legacy with the first conference even if my name was forgotten in history. This experience helped me to realize where my true passion lies and what truly matters in my career.

Nurses want to leave a mark on humanity, our patients, families, and communities. No one needs to trumpet our name, but collectively we know we are move makers who stand up for the greater good, health, and well-being of others. As a nurse, the legacy *I* want to create has an impact on my nursing colleagues.

When I left the community of NRT nurses behind (in what I hope was a better place than I found it) and moved on to become a Nurse Practitioner, I continued to serve my colleagues in my new niche by joining communities of practice for Nurse Practitioners. I stimulated discussion and helped get questions about nursing independent practice and entrepreneurship on the agendas of those who had previously given it little thought.

My schooling had left me with unanswered questions about being an NP. Questions like, "Can NPs open their own private practices in Canada? What services can we charge patients for?" I knew that if I had these questions, then other NPs had them too. Many people had told me, "No, NPs can't charge." It didn't make sense that I could only be an employee, with others making money off of my hard work.

So, I made calls and connections to seek some answers. I wanted to know if there were ways of practicing that I wasn't aware of, and of course, I discovered there were. Once I discovered that there was a false view about the services NPs could offer privately, I shared the message. Now, more and more NPs are embarking on independent practice opportunities with a new awareness of what is possible for them.

The thing about sustainability and legacy is that they aren't just about *you*. They are about the people you serve.

I want to serve my colleagues—whether that is the nursing student working as a medical secretary in my department, the bedside nurse working alongside me, the nurse educator trying to engage their staff, the nurse academic trying to disseminate their research, the nurse leader trying to lead from above, or the NP trying to move the needle in their community. I don't just want to advance *in* nursing, I want to *advance nursing*. It brings me joy, gives me energy and will be my legacy. Because it sustains me, it will be sustainable.

Legacy is an intimidating concept. As "just a nurse" you may feel that others are more equipped to build a legacy. I want to remind you that Florence Nightingale was "just a nurse" too. What made her different, was her dedication to moving the needle in the population she cared for. From improving outcomes, to tracking data, thereby proving her point in the hopes of decreasing morbidity and mortality.

Pursue your passion, plan for sustainability, make a difference, and create your legacy.

EXERCISE: Thinking about legacy

1. Who do you want to serve?
2. What is the cause you want to advance?
3. What will your legacy be?

Nursing is often about perfect action... imperfect action builds momentum.

MODULE 4

EMPOWERED: EMBRACING LIFELONG LEARNING

"But when you think about growing and being empowered yourself, it is what you've been able to do for other people that leaves you the fullest."
—Oprah Winfrey

By the end of this module, you'll know how to become empowered in your nursing career. Being empowered is about having confidence in yourself and giving yourself permission to expand your career. Knowledge, creativity, communication, resilience and embracing feedback are all components of empowerment.

NURSING EMPOWERMENT

Nursing is a challenging and rewarding career that requires compassion, knowledge, and a strong sense of responsibility. Empowerment is an essential aspect of nursing that allows you to take control of your career development.

Empowerment can take many forms, including seeking out opportunities for professional development through continuing education courses, earning advanced degrees, or obtaining certification in a specialty area. By continually learning and growing, nurses can stay current with the latest research and best practices, while improving their skills and knowledge.

Another road to empowerment is acting as an advocate for yourself and your patients. Speaking up when there are concerns about patient care and/or requesting additional resources or support is one form of advocating for others. Participating in professional organizations or groups that promote the nursing profession is another form of advocacy.

Thirdly, nurses empower themselves by taking on leadership roles within their organizations. This might involve becoming a charge nurse, leading a team, or serving on committees or boards. Leadership roles allow nurses to have a greater impact on patient care and the direction of their organizations.

STOP AND THINK

What does empowerment in your nursing career mean to you? Is there an area of your career that could benefit from empowerment?

KNOWLEDGE

In the fitness world it is common knowledge that the best type of exercise, is whatever type of exercise *you* enjoy. When we apply this lesson to education—aka brain exercise—it also means there is no one-size-fits-all approach.

Some people like running for exercise, others like dancing. Similarly, while some people love a traditional lecture, others prefer learning in small groups at a resort in the Bahamas. (What? You weren't aware that there were health professional education getaways? I can't blame you if you put down this book to Google them.) Personally, I like to study with a glass of wine in hand. I survived my Master's degree by taking my study notes to a restaurant that served alcohol, rather than sitting in a coffee shop.

When I started my career, I thought I was done learning. I thought my Bachelor's degree provided me with all of the information I needed for a successful career. I couldn't imagine investing another penny or another minute into more education, especially if there wasn't going to be a reciprocal increase in compensation. I quickly learned there is no avoiding learning in nursing.

In the first two years of my professional nursing practice, I learned time management, priority setting, strategies to deal with death and dying, how to read ECG strips, advanced wound care, IV insertion, and how to navigate relationships with colleagues on multiple units. I learned medical and surgical, cardiology, neurology, thoracic, vascular, orthopedic, gynecologic oncology, urology, and medical imaging nursing. And, just when I thought I couldn't learn anything more... I learned emergency nursing, neuro-critical care nursing, and intensive care nursing for medical-surgical, cardiac surgery, and cardiology patients.

The benefit of broad experience is that every advance in education and patient encounter taught me how *little* I actually knew. There was always more to learn. Be assured, the learning curve doesn't have to be so steep.

If you prefer a slower pace, you can climb a different mountain than the one I chose.

The early years of my career are an example of going wide—learning a broad scope in nursing. After that, I went deep, becoming more expert as I became a Nurse Practitioner and took on leadership roles. Then, when I reached—what I felt was— a pinnacle in my career I asked, "What is there to learn next?"

You may be surprised that the question "what next?" may follow you into retirement, as it did for Claudia Mariano, past president of the Nurse Practitioner Association of Ontario and author of *No One Left Behind - How Nurse Practitioners Are Changing Canada's Health Care System*. An accomplished nurse with a successful career, Mariano found that her natural inclination to look for new experiences did not cease just because she moved into the non-practicing class. She wanted to learn how to apply her expertise in new ways. Her interest in the profession, and NP practice in particular, continued to drive her.

Boredom can occur when you stop learning or because what is available for you to learn in your current area of practice doesn't interest you. If this is the case, you may experience a spike of stress hormones instead of endorphins—the good stuff!

For me, the yearly basic CPR recertification required for clinical practice represents the soul-sucking feeling of mandatory education. I have to resist the urge to roll my eyes at another round of CPR to the instructor singing "Ah-ah-ah. Staying alive! Staying alive!" I picture the instructor's blood as flooded with happy little endorphins, while *my* bloodwork would show I was half cortisol and half red blood cells.

You might have a similar feeling about some other educational prerequisite or education in general. If you're working in a role that you hate and feel you're not able to escape at this time, start thinking of your job as an opportunity to learn while getting paid. Think to yourself, "Take that administration, I'm going to get as much paid education as I can out of this crappy job!" Then start looking for opportunities to leverage the organization and grow your mind.

I promise, there is something out there that would excite you to learn. It doesn't even have to be nursing related! Maybe you would like to learn fine art appreciation, how to sing in a choir, horseback riding, sailing, or how to raise chickens.

Education does not have to be conventional. It doesn't even have to appear to relate to nursing. Many lessons can lead to transferrable skills. Your time is precious! The education you pursue has to be exciting and interesting to you. And, it has to be delivered in a way that you enjoy.

STOP AND THINK

How do you prefer to learn? Are you visual, auditory, or kinesthetic?

Think about what you have learned so far. Where can you go wider or deeper?

Share Your Knowledge

There was nothing more frustrating to me during my undergraduate and graduate studies than spending hours writing academic papers just to have them read by a teaching assistant, marked with red ink, and then never see the light of day again. It always felt like a selfish and wasteful endeavor. Practice in organized thinking as a means to gaining academic merit was a worthy objective, but *still*... frustrating. Why critically appraise and synthesize nursing literature if it will not lead to wider change?

Meanwhile, in the real world, when you write anything outside of your personal diary, there is an intended audience whose number is usually greater than one. You get to share more broadly, to deliver a message and hopefully make an impact.

Is there a topic you're interested in learning more about, but feel it would be either a waste of time or selfish? Before you begin, consider a plan to share your knowledge. This gives you a goal beyond learning for just learning's sake. When you choose your topic and envision sharing the information afterward, you build purpose and motivation for continuing education.

- *Who* will benefit from you sharing your knowledge? Patients, colleagues, government officials?
- *How* will you share with the intended audience? On social media, in an academic journal, on the 6 o'clock news?
- *When* do you want to share it? Next week, next year, posthumously?

STOP AND THINK

What will happen after you share your knowledge? Write down all the exciting outcomes that might come afterward: the thanks you will receive and the accolades.

Do you see yourself on a stage presenting to others or on the news begin interviewed? Could you write articles for the web or print? Get published in an academic journal? Do you see yourself on the road on a book tour or educating patients at the bedside?

I feel compelled to write about subjects I want to explore. Writing doesn't come easily to me, but I write to the best of my ability and I persist despite the challenge. You may not feel compelled to write a *book*, but enjoy speaking, or creating art, or sharing in less than 280 characters. It's important to choose a knowledge dissemination strategy that you enjoy and motivates you to learn—not just for learning's sake—but to provide value to others.

CREATIVITY

"**C**hocolate?" The red-nosed clown held a bedpan filled with Hershey's kisses as she made her way around our fourth-year undergraduate lecture hall. She stopped in front of the class, turned around, and introduced herself as a nurse. Not just any nurse, she was a therapeutic clown! Nursing is a creative art, but we aren't taught how to be creative in school.

In fact, nursing school can beat the creativity out of students by rewarding us when we've done something "right," and diminishing us when we've done something "wrong." Through that process, the natural inclination toward creativity is often abandoned, which is tragic.

Empowerment and creativity go hand in hand.

When nurses are empowered, we are given the freedom and autonomy to make our own decisions and take control of our own lives. This sense of control fosters creativity, innovation, and the ability to think outside the box to come up with new and unique ideas. A lack of empowerment may lead to feeling stifled, and an inability to muster creative thought.

Unlike any course I had taken previously, the last course of my Master's Degree had an option for an "aesthetic" project. The brief was to "envision and create an interpretation of the ideal primary healthcare system for the 21st century from the point of view of a healthcare stakeholder." The project could take the shape of a critical reflective narrative, poetry, collage, mobile, quilt, song, video/movie clip or documentary, picture/drawing, or sculpture. Or, instead of creating art, we could write a ten-page scholarly paper. Most of the class chose the art project.

What was surprising was how difficult this assignment was! I had written dozens of papers by that point, but never in my four years of undergraduate or two years of graduate nursing education had I ever been asked to do an art project.

My first thought was about grading. I decided my project should align with the interests of my audience - the professor marking the project. I knew she had an interest in quilting, so I thought I should make one, even though I didn't know how to work a sewing machine. Instantly, the project felt like every other twelve-point font, APA paper. Knowing that there would be a grade on my work of art immediately took away my creativity.

Become a lifelong learner outside of an academic environment, where no one is grading you. Paint for pleasure, sculpt, write a play, make an interpretive dance. Adding creativity back into your personal pursuits will give you fresh motivation to learn what was lacking in your formal education.

My creative outlet is writing. What's yours? Do you make time for it? I know I am overworking when my creative pursuits drop off. When I am struggling to move from one patient to the next, my creative mind turns off. Then, in the quiet hours in the middle of a night shift or a relatively leisurely meal break, creativity shows up again, making connections between my experiences, education, and interests. Remember, our brains are hardwired to search for ways to evolve and improve our circumstances.

We are thinking machines! When we aren't exercising our brain with creativity, reflecting, and learning our brains slowly turn off the underused areas to conserve energy. Neural connections are pruned in our sleep. We can become depressed and memory may become fuzzy.

Creativity and critical thinking are often spoken about as separate skills. Critical thinking incorporates both reason and logic. Creativity incorporates resourcefulness, imagination, and innovation. Together they enhance our problem-solving abilities.

What does creativity look like?

Sharing an idea for a better hospital unit and increased safety is the result of creative thought. The sensation of "creative wheels" turning compels us to tell stories, propose policy, and dream of the robot technology that could save the backs of our hard-working colleagues.

It took me ten years to recognize my artistic side. My focus was science for a long while; do A, get outcome B. Once you achieve expert-level knowledge, you can start to play with the science, viewing it more lightly and dissecting the necessary from the unnecessary. How freeing it is to become curious beyond the basics and to incorporate a greater number of life experiences into your nursing until one day, your scientific self has created a great work of art.

Art can be literal. The halls of Toronto General Hospital are lined with the works of Tilda Shalof, who turned thousands of brightly coloured and discarded syringe caps into grand flowing pieces of art. On the other hand, art can be subtle, as in the way you bend the reality of your sundowning Alzheimer's patient in order to help them sleep.

Practice divergent thinking to re-energize your enthusiasm for learning. Break up old ideas, make new connections, expand your limits and allow the onset of wonderful ideas.

STOP AND THINK

What creative pursuits do you enjoy? How can you bring more creativity to your nursing career?

ADVOCACY

- Are you able to speak up when a physician colleague breaks the sterile field or writes the wrong order?
- Do you contribute to conversations about short staffing as an advocate for your patients and colleagues?
- Have you confidently negotiated work contracts, asking for the salary and benefits you need to make your career sustainable?
- Would you be able to professionally say, "That's not in my job description."?

You were taught to advocate for your patients' health concerns, but it is very likely no one taught you to advocate for yourself.

Nearly every bedside nurse I have spoken with has had a complaint about workload, staffing, and safety. Why is it that I continue to hear the same thing for over a decade? Why do nurses of yesteryear recount tails of being the only nurse on a ward and going up and down the line giving medications and turning thirty patients on night shift as justification of today's nurse-to-patient ratios?

Technology has changed. The job descriptions for nurses in every area have changed. Care is more complex. There are more medications, more procedures, and more ways to keep people alive. Why are we putting up with suboptimal conditions? Fear. It's easy to vent to peers where we feel safe, but it's intimidating and scary to communicate with leaders and politicians you perceive to be higher on the ladder! The sooner you learn and practice good communication skills, the better off your career will be.

Dysfunctional communication

Nurses eat their young…and their peers, colleagues, the administration, and so on. Generally, nurses can be a difficult group of people to work with and we work in an environment of head-strong, opinionated, difficult people.

Arguably nurses have difficulty with collegiality because we are largely a female group and females typically deal with problems differently than males. We also take our role of protecting our patients, the healthcare system, society at large, and our nursing licenses very seriously. But the main reason I believe nurses are difficult is that we are an *oppressed group*.

Healthcare has a gendered history. Nursing has been seen as a largely female profession and subservient to a male-dominated profession of physicians. Nursing's resources and scope are highly limited by employers, governments, and their own professional bodies. At the same time, nurses are siloed by title and education into various nursing classes, creating a hierarchy within the profession.

Oppressed groups tend to police themselves and develop their own internal hierarchies as a means to maintain an illusion of power. They do this without even realizing it but without the right type of leaders, they tend to implode instead of directing their frustration outwards in ways that would be more productive.

Feeling powerful is a drug. Most people want to feel that they have control, and feel safe controlling members of their own rung on the hierarchy. Most nurse bullies do not even realize what they are doing. It's death by a thousand cuts. It is reflexive for them and even when confronted, they have a difficult time admitting their fault. They are just doing what was done to them.

Instead of giving power to others, realize that the only person you can truly control is yourself. You can control your thoughts and actions and where you will direct your energy. Direct your energy toward positivity, professionalism, and advocacy for your patients, yourself, and your colleagues including members of your interprofessional team.

More than one nurse has gone home and cried into their pillow, vowing never to return to the workplace because of feelings of inadequacy or mistreatment.

STOP AND THINK

What if you started keeping a journal chronicling your experiences? (Point form dates and details are enough either on paper or on your smartphone. Prefer verbal communication? Dictate to a word application.) From a scientific point of view, isn't what you are going through interesting? Wouldn't you like to know how many others have been through or are experiencing the same thing? Take note of what you feel in the moment, two hours later and the following day.

If you are in an unsafe situation, but feel too green to bring it forward—do it anyway. Confidence isn't about a lack of fear, it is about taking action *despite* it. Fearful to do it alone? Locate an ally to knock on the Chief Nursing Officer's door for you. Get yourself someone who loves to put themselves out there and recruit their natural ability to be forthcoming with opinions. You can also practice your confidence by helping a colleague advocate for themselves. There is power in numbers, even if only a mental placebo.

Assertive communication

Once you've mustered up the confidence to speak up, what do you say and how should you say it? Can you bark an order like an emergency room physician in a code? I know if I did, I would be seen more as rude rather than assertive - so for me, the answer is no. So how do you get taken seriously?

In an interview with Fotini Iconomopoulos, negotiation expert and author of *Say Less, Get More*, she said, "If you can handle a kid's temper tantrum, you can handle any negotiation with adults at work." But maybe you don't have kids, so instead, I would say, "If you can handle a sundowning patient on the night of a full moon, you can handle any negotiation with adults at work."

Start with a compliment. During my undergrad, I volunteered for a psych experiment done by a master's student. In the experiment, I took a seat at a desk and there was a female student to my right and a female student to my left. The student to my left said hello and complimented my purse, while the one on my right said hello and then remained silent. We were given a short multiple-choice test, after which the researchers questioned me about my impressions of the other students. I had a positive impression of the student who complimented me and a neutral impression of the other student. Of course, both of these students were part of the experiment. I received a copy of the results later which showed that compliments help other people to see you in a positive light. Surprise, surprise!

Add confidence. Nervous jitters? Reframe your anxiety into excitement. Do some power posing in a private space before you enter an important conversation like an interview. My personal favourite is to stand like a superhero with hands on hips, legs apart, and head up high. Don't be afraid to pause, slow down, and take a deep breath to give yourself a moment to form your thoughts.

Check your body language. Be mindful of communication not only with your words, but also your tone and body language.

Find common ground. Seek first to understand before being understood. Who are you speaking with, including their background and goals? What does the other party want?

Choose your words wisely. Know what you want to communicate and the outcome you are looking for. Avoid phrases that can cause conflict. Rather than asking "why," ask "what" or "how" to keep communication open.

Practice. My first patient encounter occurred in a lab with double-sided mirrors so that my classmates could observe as I interviewed a volunteer about their health history. High pressure, low stakes. You can practice challenging conversations in a low-pressure, low-risk environment with your peers (or teddy bears) to help you anticipate obstacles and perfect your communication skills.

Negotiation

When I graduated from my undergraduate program, contract negotiation and union politics weren't taught. The expectation was you would apply for a job, sign the contract, and get started. And, that is what I did. I spent several years with my salary increasing $0.25 a year. I very nearly reached the top of the eight-year grid where the next pay bump wouldn't occur until year 25! The ceiling of that pay structure motivated me right out of the bedside and into a master's program!

As a Nurse Practitioner student, there was an hour or two dedicated to looking at practice models with very little time dedicated to independent practice and even less to negotiating a contract. The employment contracts that were reviewed, were familiar and included: salary, benefits, education funds, vacation, and maternity leave.

When I negotiated my first independent contract as a Nurse Practitioner, I didn't have any role models to follow. I prepared by referencing the "dream job" goals that I had set for myself years before: four x 10-hour days a week, a six-figure salary, six weeks paid vacation, and maternity leave benefits. I went into the negotiation armed with a study saying NPs should be paid similarly to psychiatrists based on their level of responsibility (I still don't feel this is accurate as an NP's scope of practice is nearly as broad as a physician's) and made my ask.

Then came the offer: a contract for five days a week Monday to Friday, 8-5 pm with a salary of $40/hour as an Advanced Practice Nurse increasing to $52/hour when my Nurse Practitioner license came through (Canadian dollars and the year was 2016). There was also a promise of a year-end bonus depending on the clinic's growth.

I started negotiating back as if it were an employment contract. I asked about all of the components I had been taught to ask about. Benefits? Education funds? Vacation? The hiring manager made me feel small for asking these questions. All of the components I was asking about were for *employee* contracts, not for *contractors*.

I accepted the offer out of fear that I would lose out on the opportunity. With the promise of a year-end bonus, I convinced myself it would be worth it. Of course, the year-end bonus wasn't awarded. Based on my experience I would never accept a bonus based on a metric you can't control. Instead, negotiate the salary you want in the first place. Fotini Iconomopoulos advises, "'No' is the start of a negotiation, not the end."

That first negotiation was full of mistakes, including accepting a low offer and conceding to all the employers' requests. I didn't even talk about the hours that would work best for me. I just wanted to get my foot in the door. Sure, I got my foot in all right, but it felt wedged. I felt like I had sold my soul and was immediately dissatisfied with what I had agreed to—more hours for less than I was worth. I also set a precedent for my three-year tenure that rippled into future negotiations.

I vowed not to let others make the same mistake. Every NP student I taught as a preceptor was extensively counseled on negotiation, including what figures not to accept and why.

Unfortunately, I could not counsel prospective candidates applying to work at the clinic even though I participated in hiring and contract negotiations at the clinic. It would clearly have been a conflict of interest. All of the nurses and NPs who were hired in that three-year period had accepted even less than I had a couple of years prior and none attempted negotiation. Each time, I felt guilty as I knew the compensation was too low. Inevitably they would figure out the lesson and move on to better-paying, lower-stress positions. The take-away is that when an organization recognizes how expensive it is to lose a nurse, they will be more willing to compensate adequately.

I knew my mentorship was paying off when a candidate, who also happened to be one of my former students, came in with high salary expectations. When the counteroffer came back fifteen dollars an hour lower, she stood her ground, coming down by only fifty cents at a time and holding onto other perks she had asked for. The hiring manager finally conceded. I was proud. I never told her, but hopefully, she will read this and smile knowingly.

Ask for what you need. People want to help you. While nurses have a natural inclination to want to say yes and please others, the same can happen in reverse. There is a visceral reaction from others when we expose our vulnerability. When a puppy exposes its belly, what do you want to do? You want to give it a rub. Be vulnerable and ask. I can't promise you'll get everything you hope for in a contract negotiation but if you don't ask, the answer will always be no.

EXERCISE: Negotiation prep

1. List all of the things that would be in your ideal contract. Include: details about salary, benefits, signing bonus, relocation bonus, protected time for education, research and administration work, education funds, vacation, hours (including weekends and day or night shifts), and maternity leave.

EXPERIENCE AND RESILIENCE

I MAY BE AN ODDBALL, BUT I have been known to apply for job positions slightly outside of my area of expertise just for the experience. If I receive the opportunity to interview, I do my due diligence and research the company, the position and related subject matter in whatever depth time allows. Then, I go for it!

I once received an invitation to interview for the position of Director of Nursing Health Policy despite having no prior health policy experience. In preparation, I read Michael J. Villeneuve's *Public Policy and Canadian Nursing: Lessons from the Field* entire 407-page textbook. (Yes, I am a nerd.) By the time I finished, I felt confident that I had enough of the health policy lingo down to have a pretty convincing interview.

Ultimately, I wasn't offered the job, because I made two big mistakes in the interview. First, always research the organization—even when you think you know them well. Despite my research on nursing health policy, I forgot to refresh myself on some basic background on the organization. When put on the spot, I couldn't name even one best practice guideline from the organization despite having read several over my career. Second, always take notes during the interview. I didn't write down the instructions for the writing exercise portion of the interview, resulting in my flailing about on a blank page for thirty minutes. I laughed at myself all the way home.

My purpose wasn't to waste my time or the time of interviewers. I wanted to explore an opportunity related to my area of expertise, to see if they aligned. In the process, I gained experience. On some occasions, it also resulted in the possibility of an exciting new job opportunity. The wisdom gained through experiential learning doesn't stop with the experience itself. It extends to reflection on the experience. I didn't bomb my interview, go home and drown my sorrows, ruminating on what an idiot

I was. I learned what I would do differently for the next interview. And now, I've shared that same knowledge with you.

Of course, you can have experiences and not learn from them. You can repeat mistakes ad nauseam. As long as you aren't hurting anyone, you can make that choice. But, I promise you that not learning from your mistakes *can* hurt others; your patients and colleagues, friends and family, and your community. Everyone benefits from your self-improvement and likewise, everyone suffers from your decision to stay in limbo.

Nursing is often about perfect action

With all medical careers, perfection is the aim. To avoid medical error and catastrophic outcomes you've been trained to triple-check your work and then have a colleague triple-check what you've done. A passing grade in your nursing program was not 50%, but an 80%.

I'm asking you to throw caution to the wind and embrace a concept not taught in nursing school; imperfect action. Imperfect action is the action you can take when you're not quite ready, and don't completely know the path to reach your goal, but feel in your gut that you will eventually get there.

It's the type of action needed to get out of a rut, to put a paintbrush to a blank canvas or to let loose on the dance floor.

When you've spent several years being taught the *science* of nursing or how to do things the "right" way, then it will often appear there is only one way. Ask any nurse who has been practicing more than a year or two—there is more than one way to convince a granny to take her meds. This is the fabled and often poorly appreciated *art* of nursing.

Imperfect action builds momentum

In order to achieve a goal, you have to begin to go after it. This sounds obvious, but it is one of the most important steps in goal setting. Once you've identified a goal you have to start down the path of accomplishing it. Where do you start? Anywhere—so long as it's goal-related.

Is your first step brewing a pot of coffee, setting up your desk with fresh flowers and then taking a social media-worthy photo of your enviable office setting? Fine, but then get to work! Suddenly notice there is a load of laundry calling your name? Fine, but then get to work! Dog needs a walk? Fine, but then get to work! There will always be a thousand things to do that aren't goal-related. Prioritize your goal by dedicating time to imperfect action to get you going.

Finally having your butt in the chair, or hitting the enroll button on that program you've been researching or even starting that e-mail to a former mentor counts as action you know can propel you forward. You just have to find a way to stay motivated.

There will be mental blocks to overcome. Your air conditioning will inevitably go on the fritz and your favourite pen will run out of ink. That's ok. You're not aiming for perfection in the beginning, just action. With every problem solved, you will become mentally tougher and more resilient in the pursuit of your goals.

Resilience is the ability to take a hit, and bounce back. Pre-2020, working understaffed and being floated to unfamiliar floors was not the norm unless you were a member of a float pool or Nursing Resource Team. Having started my career in a Nursing Resource Team, I became resilient from the get-go. This paid off for one of my former Resource Team colleagues who worked in the ER during the craziness of 2020-2022 where she saw many coworkers leave nursing altogether. She and her colleagues all experienced the same chaos and the same short staffing. Having acquired—not only a thick skin but an elastic one—paid off when times got tough. For Resource Team nurses, the word resilience is a mantra, a positive trait or virtue developed by working in understaffed units where the unit nurses (while doubting your competence) dumped the most challenging workloads on you. We are all born with the capacity to be resilient, but it takes uncertainty and hardship to unlock it as a trait.

When you first start working toward a goal it might feel easy. Initially, you have fresh motivation, but the middle part is where complacency lives.

Your willpower may fail you. You will need resilience to push through to the end. In tough points of my career, I take pressure off by telling myself - this isn't my *life's work*, this is *work*. Somehow taking the adjective away frees me up to continue on, no matter how imperfectly.

Nobody cares about the foot care business you've thought about starting, or the academic article you wrote halfway and then put on the shelf. They want to know about the business you've opened or the research you've published! They want to know about what you've finished!

Your success is not in your ability to start a goal or project but in your ability to complete one—perfect or not. When I applied to graduate school I thought about the worst-case scenarios,

- What if I don't get in? Well, I'll still have my nursing license.
- What if I fail or drop out? Well, I'll still have my nursing license.
- What if I graduate and don't like my career as a Nurse Practitioner? Well, I'll still have my nursing license.
- What if I lose my nursing license while I'm in school? Well, I'll still have my nursing experience.
- What if I can't get a permanent job after giving up my comfortable hospital nursing salary and benefits? Well, I'll have to work casual hours.
- What if I don't apply to graduate school at all? Well, you will always wonder if you should have applied.

Any "bad" outcome was better than feeling regret.

I delayed applying to graduate school for two years longer than I needed to. I delayed writing this book for years. I didn't brag about the book I was thinking about writing for five years, but you had better believe I am bragging about publishing this book, whether or not anyone actually reads or likes it!

Nothing is ever finished with a first draft. There are always corrections and edits, but there is no opportunity for improvement without first finishing the work.

You might fail. A lot of people fail tests. Businesses fail and people go bankrupt. What makes you so special that you are not allowed to fail? More than one nurse I know failed their licensing exams one or more times!

Give yourself an "A" for effort. Few people make it to goal completion. If you do, then you will be ahead—even if you don't get the outcome you were hoping for! You will learn more from failing than you will from not trying.

STOP AND THINK

What is an example of an imperfect action you've taken in your life and what was the outcome? What have you been putting off finishing?

EMBRACE FEEDBACK

We don't know what we don't know. Sometimes, we don't *want* to know what we don't know. Ignorance is bliss.

Often, others are able to see things that we can't see about ourselves. If you're in a rut and not sure where to start in your learning journey and pursuit of nursing career success, try looking outside of yourself for input.

Feedback can be scary because we often associate it with criticism but, the right type of feedback can be a building block to your success. Constructive feedback is supportive. Instead of only highlighting strengths and weaknesses, it also focuses on solutions and next steps. Feedback doesn't have to be formal or intimidating. Informal feedback can be received on a regular basis through constructive conversations.

When I dipped my toes into project management, it wasn't because I wanted to get into project management, it was the result of constructive feedback. In a hallway conversation, my unit nurse educator suggested I apply to a new nursing research and fellowship program being offered at my hospital. She felt it would be a good opportunity to grow my leadership skills. I never would have considered applying if it wasn't for her. She saw potential in me that wasn't on my radar. Similarly, when I became a clinic director, it wasn't because I applied, it was because a physician colleague recommended it to me in conversation.

Oftentimes we get unsolicited feedback, but don't overlook opportunities to ask for feedback. Consider the title of Ryan Holiday's book, *The Obstacle is the Way*. When feedback comes, try not to get your back up or be offended. Pretend you have a thick skin or protective bubble around you, and slowly resilience will set in.

Unsolicited feedback is often either all or nothing. You are either getting five-star or one-star reviews, but not much in between. Meanwhile, the most useful feedback are those three-star reviews that are more likely an honest critique, sharing both positives (strengths) and negatives (areas to improve on).

While it strokes the ego to hear you're perfect, you actually *want* some three-star reviews. Approach colleagues (not your typical break buddy) to provide honest feedback, and tell them you're not looking for a five-star review. Let them know you are open to constructive feedback and are looking for areas of improvement. If you don't feel comfortable doing this yourself, get a third party involved. Ask a friend or manager to pick three colleagues to provide anonymous feedback and return the results to you in a sealed envelope.

This type of feedback is going to help you to understand what others consider to be your strengths and where areas for improvement exist. You can pursue opportunities that make use of your strengths, while reflecting on, and addressing your weaknesses. You don't have to agree with all of the feedback. Focus on areas that appeal to you.

A note about feedback; never take offense. Sometimes the feedback is less about you, and more about the person providing it. Some people are not skilled at giving feedback and instead of providing something constructive, they will unintentionally (or intentionally) deliver feedback in a way that can make you feel like crawling into a hospital bed and eating red Jell-O for the rest of your days. Whenever someone says something that sounds hurtful, bite your tongue. Take a breath and think about the intention behind the words. The only person you can control is you. If someone says something malicious, don't give them the satisfaction. Perhaps they are having a rough day, or are honestly clueless about effective communication.

Once you have solicited feedback, you can return to the first module and set yourself new, relevant goals. Reevaluate once a year or whenever you're in a rut and not making the progress in your career that you would like to.

EXERCISE: Feedback helps!

1. Identify three people to ask for constructive feedback about you as an individual or professional.

2. What feedback will you act on?

You are uniquely talented and
qualified with
unlimited potential.

MODULE 5

BUILDING A CAREER WITHOUT LIMITS!

"If you embrace that the things that you can do are limitless, you can put your ding in the universe. You can change the world."

—Tim Cook

By the end of Module 5 you will have identified and overcome the limiting beliefs that have been holding you back from the successful nursing career you desire. For many, limiting beliefs have been built over a lifetime. As a nursing professional, it's time to question their validity and create changes where your belief system is not serving you. To figure out how to create a limitless career, let's start by exploring what limiting beliefs are, and then identify the beliefs that commonly show up in nursing.

LIMITING BELIEFS IN NURSING

You might be thinking, "I'm just like everyone else. There is nothing special about me. Nothing deserving of an exceptional nursing career. I'm the "do my time and get out" type. I couldn't possibly be a leader or teacher or business owner or public speaker or writer or any other thing besides what I am now. Financial rewards and recognition are for other people, not for me!"

Au contraire, my friend! You *are* uniquely talented and qualified with unlimited potential. If you made it this far in life, you can make it anywhere you want to go, so long as you get out of your own way!

STOP AND THINK

What would you do with your career, if money was no object and you had unwavering support?

How do you feel about the following statements:

- I'm *just* a nurse.
- Developing expertise is above my pay grade. Nurses shouldn't advertise or make sales because it's too braggy and sleazy.
- Nurses shouldn't work independently of doctors.
- Nurses are employees, not business owners.
- Nurses making a six-figure salary are working a lot of shift work and overtime.
- Nurses shouldn't be millionaires.
- Nursing is hard and I just have to accept it and work harder.
- Nurse managers have no idea how hard nursing is and should put their scrubs back on and help out.

- Nurses are passionate about nursing and that should be enough compensation.
- I would pursue my passion, but only for the quirky nurses and I'm not quirky.
- Nurses are too nice to be CEOs.
- Nurses are nice, normal people and nice normal people don't have passion.

Did you agree with the statements? Did they make you cringe?

Limiting beliefs are thoughts or opinions you believe to be true that prevent you from moving forward in your personal or professional life. You may have learned your limiting beliefs related to the nursing profession from your family, the media, your education, your employer, your patients, or your peers. In many cases, we absorb these beliefs by osmosis in our nursing education and the early parts of our careers. You may also have experienced trauma or other difficult-to-process events which led to creating boundaries that were once protective but have become overly limiting. Limiting beliefs can creep in unexpectedly and are often only revealed with close examination.

Limiting beliefs make you feel the need to ask for permission before you envision or pursue a goal. Unfortunately, waiting for the world to grant you permission is a waste of time and energy. You can have more than what you believe you can—right now—by moving the goalpost of your beliefs or even removing them altogether.

Imagine you had a child who said, "When I grow up, I want to be the first nurse astronaut on Mars. It's my dream!" What would you say to that child? Do you remember a time when you were told "no" you couldn't be that thing you wanted to be? Are you going to repeat the pattern of your childhood and tell them to lower their expectations and choose something less risky or more profitable? Or, are you going to tell them they can be, and do, anything? Now, let's give that child a name— "your inner child."

In nursing, limiting beliefs can take many forms and be related to a variety of issues, such as:

1. Professional development: the belief that you are not qualified or capable of taking on new challenges or responsibilities, such as earning an advanced degree or becoming a leader in your organization.

2. Patient care: the belief that you are not capable of making a positive impact on patient care, or that your efforts are not valued or appreciated by others.

3. Self-worth: the belief that you are not worthy of respect or recognition from colleagues or superiors, or that you are not deserving of professional advancement or success.

4. Workplace culture: the belief that your organization is not supportive of professional development or that there are barriers to advancement that cannot be overcome.

One of my personal limiting beliefs emerged two years into my nursing career when I was working in the ER of a busy downtown hospital. After a 12-hour shift, a handful of colleagues and I would go to a diner for breakfast or to a dive bar for nachos and drinks. I had a new boyfriend who I was really smitten with and fit my ideal prototype for husband material. A few months into our relationship I casually mentioned these after-work hangouts. He replied, "It's strange to go out with coworkers after work. You should really stop doing that." I was convinced he was right, and stopped going out after work. After a week or two of declining invites after work, I called up my best friend and asked her if I had been in the wrong. She told me I needed to break up with the schmuck I was dating and gave me a word for the type of abuse he was dishing out—*gaslighting*. My ex's claim wasn't outrageous and didn't hurt me in any obvious way, but he created a false narrative that prevented me from networking with my peers in a completely normal and healthy way.

Gaslighting doesn't only show up in personal relationships, I've also experienced it from colleagues, managers, employers, and during contract negotiations for jobs I didn't even have yet—big red flag. I've even experienced gaslighting from myself—*self-gaslighting*. I've been made to feel like my facts were false, I've had my ideas stolen and presented as someone else's, and I've been made to feel like an imposter. Now that I recognize gaslighting and its negative effect, I combat it with awareness and assertiveness. A couple of examples — "I agree that *my* idea to implement a follow-up system will benefit patients;" "I see that your perspective is different from *mine*. I respectfully disagree," and "I deserve support for the things I've achieved and to be taken seriously." Learn from my experience and don't accept gaslighting from anyone, especially yourself!

We can't change limiting beliefs unless we are aware of them

Pay attention to the language you use in regards to nursing, your career, and your money. When you make an absolute statement like, "I can't" or "nurses don't," ask yourself, is it really impossible? And, is this statement true? When your gut tells you something is not quite right, seek a second opinion—perhaps even a third opinion from someone like a therapist who will have an unbiased opinion.

It's time to explore and smash some limiting beliefs that might be holding you back in your career. I believe in you! You can do it!

EXERCISE: Limiting beliefs

1. Write down three limiting beliefs that are holding you back. Not sure you have any? *Return* to this question at the end of the chapter.

NURSING INCOME BELIEFS

When nurses renew their annual nursing college registration, the question is asked—"Have you practiced nursing in the past year?"

Nurses on *maternity leave* who've been caring for a newborn and a three-year-old using nursing knowledge, skill, and judgment ask themselves, "Am I practicing nursing?"

Nurses on *family leave* who've been caring for aging parents—one of whom has dementia and the other who recently experienced a stroke—ask themselves, "Am I practicing nursing?"

Attempts made by nursing colleges to justify who should, or shouldn't be, included in the "practicing class" of nursing are fraught with contradictions. I can promise you, I learned more about maternal and infant nursing from going through pregnancy, childbirth, and the first twelve months of motherhood, than I ever learned in undergraduate or graduate school! Yet, caring for loved ones doesn't count as nursing. Paid care for strangers using the same knowledge, skill and judgment *does* count. Why is that? Because nursing is a profession—a *paid* occupation.

Family caregiving, unpaid work, and volunteer work does not always count in the eyes of nursing colleges, no matter how skilled you may be in those activities.

Nursing compensation

Are you already uncomfortable at the thought of contemplating your salary? Join the crowd. Many nurses have learned that money is not something to talk about or ask for more of.

Nurses have been socialized to have guilt around wanting more money, (possibly from the very beginning) because nursing was associated with religious service. In the formative years of nursing, hours were long and wages were low. As nursing has evolved, the pay and hours have improved, but inequity persists.

Sex-based inequity is a clear issue in modern professional nursing both within and outside of the profession. As far back as the 1920s, there is evidence of sex-based inequity with male nurses making more than female nurses. It's an issue that is complex and multifactorial. While women continue to comprise a majority of the nursing workforce, men generally earn higher salaries. Although there has been some progress in reducing the nursing pay gap in recent years, income disparities persist.

In some respects, this isn't a surprise. Men are socialized to be the breadwinners, to negotiate higher salaries and to ask for, and expect, raises. Also, when comparing nursing to other publicly-funded professions like policing and firefighting, we see that male-dominated professions earn more and get higher raises year-over-year. Inequity increases and moving the needle on the issue is painfully slow.

The mental block around money gets ugly when nurses decide to dip their toes into private practice. Many nurses have trouble thinking about charging for their services. Charging a "hospital" an hourly rate is easy because there is usually a union bargaining on behalf of the nurse. This leaves the money talks distanced from the individual nurse, and moral distress is generally averted. At the same time, offering private services to a 97-year-old widow who is counting dimes out of her purse can cause mixed feelings.

If you work with marginalized populations, you may feel that nurses are exceedingly affluent and selfish for wanting more money when it could go to programs for those less fortunate. But, let's be honest—whether paid by public or private dollars—there are executives, doctors, lawyers, and psychologists working with the same populations who make more money than nurses, and still sleep soundly at night.

How many times have you made this calculation? One Saturday night shift (aka base pay per hour multiplied by 1.5 plus one dollar an hour weekend bonus over 12 hours) equals one-twelfth of a trip to the Bahamas for five days.

No questions are raised on the morality of charging more for services after 40 hours of shift work— even though it requires the same knowledge, skill, and judgment. In fact, many nurses *seek out* overtime to raise their bottom line! Canadian nurses want to reach the threshold for Canada's "sunshine list" that identifies/exposes public servants who make more than $100K.

STOP AND THINK

Do you fantasize about winning the lottery and handing in your resignation when you get that big windfall? Can you think of that one nurse who would keep nursing afterward, despite their newfound millionaire status? What would you do? Donate a portion of the money to charity? Feel guilty about those who didn't play the workplace lottery pool that week and decide to share the winnings with them?

We all need money to pay for food, the roof over our head, cell phone bills, medications, supporting our children or parents or partners, and yes—for taking a well-deserved vacation!

As a unionized nurse, you may have an opinion about the pay scale, but you likely accept the stepwise increases, and look forward to your yearly pay bump. You may also lament that the extra $0.50 per hour this year hasn't affected your bottom line as it is barely keeping up with inflation.

Nurses make up a substantial part of the healthcare workforce. Hospital boards and governments bemoan giving nurses raises because a small raise across the board leads to significant costs to the bottom line. Nursing positions are also frequently the first to be slashed in the name of budget balancing. The general population ultimately suffers in the form of poorer healthcare outcomes, but the cycle of adding and cutting nursing positions in hospitals, long-term care homes and other sectors persists.

Nurse Practitioners in Ontario are one of the best examples of nurses' inability to recognize and advocate for their worth. I love my colleagues, but this has to be addressed. Nurse Practitioners in Ontario promote themselves as a group who can help meet the needs of individuals without family physicians or who live in low-income or rural populations, at a cost that is far cheaper than physicians.

What they *should* have been addressing with the Ontario government, is that Nurse Practitioners are being paid less than Registered Nurses. In what other profession does your wage go down when your education and responsibilities go up?

When I entered the Nurse Practitioner program in 2014, I was shocked to learn Nurse Practitioners in Primary Health Care had been on a pay freeze for six years—putting their salaries *below* that of their Registered Nurse counterparts in the hospital, despite more years of education and more risks and responsibilities on their licenses. At such a low wage it was no wonder that recruitment and retention of Nurse Practitioners was a problem. I am still surprised Nurse Practitioners were agreeing to practice at all!

In 2020, during the pandemic, individual Nurse Practitioners surprised me again by saying they would volunteer to work with the NHL on COVID-19 nasal swab duty. The argument couldn't be made that the NHL was a low-income or small business! The NHL didn't need volunteers, though I'm sure they happily accepted free labor.

Those tip-toeing into "independent practice" are also guilty of money sabotage. Here is how one nurse described their fee for a house call service on an online forum:

> "It's a flat fee to visit someone in their home. Another service referenced in this post is a bit of a bigger business so they charge different rates depending on what is needed. I am doing this

more as a service to those without primary care providers while they are waiting to be rostered. The waitlist is quite long for primary care here. I just charge a flat fee. Should be noted, this is an after-hours service for me; I have a full-time job, so this is not a money-making project. The other business' website though has been quite informative as I was setting up this business."

I looked up their service fees and found they were charging $30 Cdn for a house call, or $45 for an "extended" house call. $30 for a 30-minute home visit is not as simple as it sounds.

A home visit used to be the norm for healthcare providers. Now, a home visit is really a premium service. The nurse in this forum knew she was undercharging, stating their services were not intended to make money because they already had a full-time job!

You might be thinking they *are* making money. $45 per half hour is equivalent to $90 per hour, right? That's $180,000 a year full-time! That sounds like a pretty good wage. No, not at all. Let's break it down further.

A nurse working part-time or casual hours in addition to their full-time job needs to pay to maintain: a website, a car, a home office including a computer, a cell phone, business insurance, and supplies like masks, gloves, and hand sanitizer. This same nurse may also need a receptionist or virtual assistant to answer requests for service and to schedule visits. A return trip to someone's home can take anywhere from ten to thirty minutes or more in each direction. There is time required for booking and confirmation of a patient visit, and additional paperwork after it's completed. What about the cost of cancellations? In the end, there is a good chance the nurse was actually *losing* money! Your business is not a business if you are not making money! It is a hobby or volunteering.

The previous example was an NP providing service from the goodness of their heart. The payment was not monetary, instead, it was in the good feelings they received from helping others. This nurse saw an unmet need and stepped up to provide service for little to no profit, taking time away from writing a memoir or spending time with family, or some other "selfish" pursuit.

However altruistic this may seem; this type of pricing sets a precedent in the marketplace—NP home visits for a bargain price! I can only assume that this nurse got their pricing strategy from a physician colleague who offers home visits, but forgot that physicians can charge provincial health insurance on top of the private fee.

As a Nurse Practitioner, I struggled to describe myself as anything but a nurse with the responsibilities of a doctor. The reality is that a Nurse Practitioner does much of the same assessment, diagnosis, and treatment as a physician with fewer differences in scope as time goes on. Despite this, as I've already pointed out, the salary is far closer to that of a Registered Nurse. For this reason, many Nurse Practitioners freely fail to renew their designation.

Knowing this early on, I set out to ask for my worth in salary negotiations and to charge my worth for one-on-one consultations with patients or colleagues seeking advice. Some nurse colleagues were offended, thinking "advice" should be free, but anyone who paid my fee told me by the end of the consultation that they would gladly pay again. I have only so many hours in the day, so if I am to take time away from my family, I need to offset lost time with compensation.

A career is not viable if it is not financially sustaining you. Repeat it with me. *A career is not viable if it is not financially sustaining you!*

Frequently, nurses leave the profession because the responsibilities of the job and compensation are not in alignment. What if you really don't want to leave nursing, preferring to use your skills to impact population health and wellness?

The first thing you need to do is get rid of your money paradigm and make a shift! Do you think the CEO of your local hospital is greedy and overpaid? Do you think your physician colleagues are stuck-up because they make three times your salary? Do you think that a six-figure salary is unattainable for you? How much is your time worth an hour? Fifteen dollars? Thirty? Seventy-five? One hundred? Two hundred? Five hundred? One thousand?

I worked minimum wage jobs from the age of fifteen. In my first job in 2003, I earned $6.85 an hour. Looking back, I wouldn't have believed that I would grow up to charge over ten times that amount, never mind twenty or over thirty times that an hour. When I started my own business, it was a challenge to figure out an hourly rate. I had to get over my poverty mindset, and become comfortable with the idea that money is fluid and abundant.

Money is a message, a language, and a currency. It is not good or bad. Your ethics and self-worth are not a reflection of the number in your bank account. The amount of money you are offered may not be directly in line with the value you bring. In fact, the work of nurses is *so* valuable that hospital-employed nurses are deemed an essential service![10]

A nursing wage in Canada is more or less standardized to reflect the need to control the nursing workforce and the provinces' budgets. A fully employed nurse makes what most would consider a good living. However, a ceiling on salary is not a ceiling on earning *potential*.

When you are thinking about your future career, you also have to think about money. No nurse should be working for free. The hours you spend reporting or finishing charts or helping to turn a patient one last time after your shift, are unpaid "volunteer" hours. Historically nursing has been a volunteer position, but not today.

The extra hours you are putting in for free could be spent with family, on personal or professional development, on self-care, or a side business. If you work twelve hours—which we all know is more like thirteen hours—and also spend an hour commuting to your workplace, you can't

---

10 In Canada, an essential service is defined as a service, facility, or activity that is or will be, at any time, necessary for the safety or security of the public or a segment of the public. As such, nurses in hospitals and long-term care facilities are deemed essential and cannot strike, taking away their power to demand equitable compensation.

squeeze eight hours of sleep, meal preparation, family time, exercise, meditation, and so on into the rest of your day. Helping a colleague may feel nice, but you are doing a disservice to yourself, to your colleagues, and to your patients. They deserve safe staffing levels instead of you burning out or injuring yourself.

STOP AND THINK

If you are currently putting in extra hours your first piece of homework is to start documenting your time. How much extra (unpaid) time are you putting in a day? How quickly does it add up in a week? A month? You might be shocked by the numbers.

Now, multiply your number by your hourly rate. How much money are you losing out on? 3 hours a week for 52 weeks is in the thousands of dollars. Have you already rationalized the loss by thinking you wouldn't be able to do anything else with those extra hours? You wouldn't be able to make money in the hour after your full-time job, so the money isn't really lost?

I am telling you that you could make money in that time! Running CPR classes, tutoring nursing students, teaching resume writing, or running a post-shift meditation class, are just a few creative examples to supplement your salary in the hour after work.

Unlike money, time is a resource we can get back. We can only spend time. Spend your time wisely. Advocate for yourself. Don't wait for retirement.

Options for extra income

First, consider who will pay you. Payment can be put into two categories:

   a. *Private funds* come from individuals, corporations, or insurance companies. For example, an individual hiring a nurse privately for foot care, a nurse being contracted privately by a corporation for employee wellness, legal nurse consulting or being hired by a private for-profit corporation.

b. *Public funds* come from municipal, provincial, or national level funding. For example, in Canada, nurses are commonly employed by public hospitals or public health organizations.

Income-earning relationships may be as an employee, a contractor, or a consultant.

When you think about your ideal career, you want to be able to define your goal income and ideal payment model. Working in a public hospital comes with perks like benefits and a pension. Conversely, a contractor or consultant has to self-invest in benefits and savings. These are important considerations, as benefits and pension contributions can account for up to 20% above your base salary.

If you are considering leaving a full-time role, it is important to calculate the equivalent needed to make your career financially sustainable.

EXERCISE: Income goals

1. What is the ceiling of your nursing income if nothing changes?
2. How do you feel about your nursing income?
3. Will making more money as a nurse make you feel bad? Why or why not?
4. What is your income goal? How can you get there?

NURSING STATUS BELIEFS

I NEVER WANT TO HEAR THE phrase "I'm *just* a nurse" ever again. Humility is a virtue, but there is such a thing as being too humble. "Just a nurse" is *just an excuse* to play small and downplay your accomplishments and it can become part of your self-image.

Where does this phrase come from? You don't hear a gerontologist, neurosurgeon, or cardiologist saying, "I'm *just* a doctor." Nursing has a nuanced history that has traditionally placed the nurse in a subservient role whether to a physician or to God. Rightfully, values including altruism, autonomy, human dignity, integrity, honesty, and social justice are largely reinforced by the nursing curriculum. Let's examine that first word. Altruism.

Altruism means showing a selfless concern for the well-being of others. This means putting the needs of *everyone* else before *yourself*. In emergency situations, for short periods of time, altruism can be necessary and reasonable. I will never forget the February 2022 war image of Ukraine nurses crammed into a makeshift bomb shelter, caring for NICU babies. On cots wrapped in blankets, one nurse calmly bagged a preemie. These are extreme measures for extraordinary times. If, under normal circumstances, you are ignoring your needs for those of your patients, you will eventually be left with nothing to give.

Consider the impact of chronic understaffing. If a unit is occasionally understaffed, it can be reasonable to forgo your needs for a brief period if you are otherwise healthy and adequately recognized for your additional efforts. The problem is that understaffing has been used to balance budgets since before I began my nursing career in 2008. The hospitals I worked at regularly ran above 100% capacity. I heard over and over again that beds in the hallways of the emergency department were temporary, but over ten years later they had become fixtures. I suffered for my patients and profession—largely accepting a status quo of no breaks, but

I now know I was being taken advantage of by a system that depends on nurses' value of altruism and of our lives being *less valuable than* others.

As a clever alternative to "I'm just a nurse," I used to say "that's beyond my pay grade." Manage the unit when the charge nurse calls in sick? That's beyond my pay grade. Be able to read an x-ray? That's beyond my pay grade. Take on any extra responsibility that could propel my career forward? That's beyond my pay grade! Wait…what? Why wouldn't I want to expand my horizons? Because, I was scared and wanted to protect myself from failure.

No matter what way you say it, when you downplay your value and your abilities it causes you to be underestimated. When you believe you're *just* a nurse you are underestimating yourself. Your work may go unnoticed and you may even reject accolades when they come your way. You will not be able to evolve your career or become a leader with this mindset.

After organizing the Nurse Resource Teams conference, I came up with a theory on the needs of nurses in organized float pools. This theory extends to most nurses, but became obvious to me after sitting in a room with 100 nurses who were used to being nomads in their respective hospitals.

The theory was based on Maslow's Hierarchy of needs, introduced in Module 1. You may recall that in Maslow's Hierarchy, basic human needs like food, water, and shelter must be met before someone can reach self-actualization and full potential. Many nurses at the conference were expressing a desire to have basic needs met; things like coverage to use the washroom and a secure place to store their belongings. These seemingly basic gripes prevented us from diving deeper into matters of patient safety and the goal of feeling professionally fulfilled in their roles.

In hopes of moving the needle on the basic needs front, I shared my theory with the nursing leadership of the hospital. Instead of offering up funding and space for lockers, the response from leadership was, "Are you going to publish this?"

I was thrown off by the question. Here I was, standing in front of them as *just a nurse* who wanted some lockers for my colleagues. Instead, they were reflecting back at me that I was a leader with the potential to put my observations into print. I walked in feeling low on the totem pole and my ego wasn't ready for their response. I became overwhelmed and never went on to publish the findings from the conference because I wasn't ready to evolve beyond a limited view of myself.

I was weighed down by imposter syndrome despite my significant professional accomplishments. I felt I was still in the trenches, hoping for a locker of my own and didn't yet see that I could also occupy the ranks of leadership. Imposter syndrome takes the form of a voice saying, "I'm in over my head and they're going to find out!"

What did I learn by reflecting on this experience? You have to recognize and meet your basic needs before you will give yourself permission to go bigger.

STOP AND THINK

Nurses work with physicians, respiratory therapists, social workers, chiropractors, naturopaths, personal support workers, patients, the CEO, and others. Did you immediately place yourself in a hierarchy amongst the list? Did reading some of those professions evoke an emotion for you? Maybe you really dislike CEOs or feel naturopaths aren't real doctors. Of what benefit to your career is it to rank yourself among these other groups? What is the benefit/cost if you judge others harshly? What could you gain by seeing all of these players as equals?

THE BUSINESS OF NURSING

Have you ever convinced a patient to take their morning stool softener? Congratulations, you're in sales! Even if you aren't making a cash transaction with your patient, you *are* being paid for your time and expertise by your employer. If you're practicing in the public system in Canada, you don't think about the cost of medications or your time providing nursing services because they are paid by taxes rather than the individual at the point of care. Meanwhile, if you are in private practice or practice as a nurse outside of Canada, patients are charged for every tablet taken and gauze pad used.

Now that you see you are in medical "sales," how do you reconcile that with your career? How can you sell your services, professional advice, medical devices, and pharmaceuticals and then make money and not feel icky about it?

Let's start with traditional employment such as nursing in a hospital or nursing home. Negotiating an employment contract is an exercise in sales. You sold your employer on hiring you for a specific price, for a specific number of hours of your time and they pay you according to that agreement. Before you signed your contract, did you negotiate the price or take the price offered? Were your services "on-sale" because you were in need of money or experience immediately? Or, did you charge a premium for your years of experience and positive patient outcomes?

Next, consider private practice as a solo practitioner, contractor, or consultant. What about being an entrepreneur who builds a business with employees, such as medical aesthetics or a staffing agency. Have you thought of these as possibilities for yourself? Are you held back by the thought of commanding your own prices?

Author and former nurse, Melane Mullings, built and sold a staffing agency. Motivated by the less-than-ideal care she had received as a patient, she described building the business one conversation at a time.

She identified an area of need, told her story of being on the receiving end of suboptimal care, and got buy-in from other people interested in supporting her cause. No sleazy sales tactics, just an honest pitch that resonated with others. She made an impact on rural nursing staffing. The money followed.

STOP AND THINK

Contract nurses (such as travel nurses) typically make more per hour than traditionally employed nurses. How do you feel about staffing agencies, knowing how much their nurses make for their contracts and that the business has to make a profit on top of that?

People underestimate the money required to run a business, or to plan for unstable employment. Being so used to receiving a salary, we forget about things like overhead and profits, and costs for simple things like printer paper to more intimidating lawyer fees. Do you start to see how these numbers add up? Anyone saying these nurses or agencies are greedy just isn't seeing the bigger picture because yes, you are allowed to make a margin of profit above your salary and expenses!

What about nurses who actually are *in* sales? Nurses make ideal candidates to sell medical equipment or to be pharmaceutical reps. We understand the patient, the provider, and the science. How do you feel about these nurses? Have they "sold their soul" and are taking advantage of innocent people in need? Or are they being of service by helping to bring options to market?

Most nursing schools don't offer a Business 101 course, but related skills are embedded in our education. Instead of "sales and marketing" we "build rapport and trust" or instead of "CEO" we use "critical thinking, prioritizing, organization, and managing emergencies." We aren't given examples of CEOs whose credentials include RPN or RN and, we certainly aren't taught to be the CEO of our own credentials!

What I hope you take away from this section, is that nurses have all of the transferable skills necessary to run a business and make sales. and you can expand this skillset into countless areas. Don't let other people tell you that nurses can't make sales or run a business. You have my permission to venture outside of the norm!

EXERCISE: The business of nursing

1. What skills do you have that are transferable to running your own business?
2. How do you feel about making sales?
3. Do a web search for "successful nurse entrepreneurs" and be inspired.

IMPOSTER SYNDROME AND FEAR OF FAILURE

I ONCE READ IN AN EMERGENCY department physician's consult note, *"heroically prescribed patient Aspirin."* Call it ego or cheekiness—we have all encountered those who don't appear to suffer from a lack of confidence. Yet research say that as many as 82% of high-achieving individuals experience imposter syndrome and feel like a phony despite their accomplishments, at some point in their careers.[11]

Have you ever noticed the documentation of a physician versus a nurse? It is one confidently scribbled line versus pages of prose written with crippling perfectionism. Nurses will fearfully write pages of documentation in case they are called to court and have to prove they wiped the patient front to back and not back to front. The typical legal advice nurses hear is to "chart as much as possible." On the other hand, I've also been advised that the more you chart the more room there is for criticism.

I'm not giving legal advice but do want to point out that nurses have a hard time knowing what is "good enough" and this can be reflected in the way we view ourselves. Can you ever be a "good enough" nurse? One who gives the right amount of care, attention, time, and energy and has the right amount of expertise? Not if your psyche doesn't allow you to see yourself as "good enough" and is steeped in fear of failure.

Imposter syndrome

On a message board for nurses one poster asked, "Any tips/tricks/suggestions for overcoming imposter syndrome? Five years as a nurse and it's

---

11 Bravata, D. M., Watts, S. A., Keefer, A. L., Madhusudhan, D. K., Taylor, K. T., Clark, D. M., Nelson, R. S., Cokley, K. O., & Hagg, H. K. (2020). Prevalence, Predictors, and Treatment of Impostor Syndrome: A Systematic Review. *Journal of general internal medicine*, 35(4), 1252–1275. Retrieved from https://doi.org/10.1007/s11606-019-05364-1

the worst it's been." Within hours there were over fifty responses.

"Eleven years in, and it still happens!!"

"20 years in, and still happens."

"22 years and I'm still questioning myself."

"9 years and still going strong."

"I've been feeling less and less confident as time goes by...graduated 7 years ago and feel much less competent now than I did then."

I asked myself, "What is imposter syndrome exactly? Why is it persisting in expert-level nurses? And, how can I help them?!"

What I discovered was that imposter syndrome is a psychological phenomenon whereby individuals doubt their accomplishments and feel like they are not qualified or capable of their success. It is a common experience and can affect people from all walks of life, including professionals in fields such as nursing. It is important for individuals to recognize and address imposter syndrome in order to achieve their full potential.

I wasn't an "imposter syndrome" expert—aside from my own experiences— but I moved quickly because I saw a need and knew enough to get started. That day, I advertised a workshop titled "Overcoming Imposter Syndrome." I registered 15 nurses, ranging from student to expert, and a week later the session was a success. The opportunity to come together, learn strategies, hear each other's experiences and provide impartial feedback was reassuring.

I started by sharing my experiences with imposter syndrome in different stages and areas of my career, imposter syndrome as a bedside nurse, educator, and leader. For example, when I was offered the role of Clinic Director, I initially felt that they only chose me because no one else applied. Meanwhile, the reality was that I was really good at my job, my patients liked me, and my leadership potential was recognized. I earned that position.

Participants also shared their experiences with imposter syndrome. One participant voiced, "I have an incredible amount of stress in my job, feel constantly pushed out of my comfort zone without enough time to get comfortable or master things. My boss just quit, so I will be taking on part of that role on top of my usual work. I combat my feelings of self-doubt by working ALL the time (day, night, and weekends)."

To combat imposter syndrome, I shared five strategies:

1. *Build a support system.* Your support system can give you affirmation—reminding you that you are talented and smart—and accountability. They can remind you of your goals and that you should be pursuing them.
2. *Self-affirmation.* Remind yourself of your strengths and successes. Yes, you have both of these!
3. *Build effective rituals.* I recommend starting your day on a positive note by planning ahead, logging accomplishments, and building in time for reflection.
4. *Reframe negative thoughts.* Disrupt the cycle of "trigger, negative thought, negative feeling, self-sabotaging action" by recognizing your negative thought and making it neutral or positive.
5. *Acceptance.* Accept that perfection is unrealistic and that you're supposed to feel discomfort in times when you need to develop new competencies. You are supposed to feel out of your depth or challenged so that you can grow.

Think back to nursing school when you had an exam where your answer was correct, but marked as wrong. This is an example of a professional—a nursing professor—putting out imperfect work. Did you point your finger and say, "Aha! I have found you out! You are no professor, but a fraud!" No, it was annoying but you got over it, got the pass you needed and the professor's tenure was never questioned.

We are all imperfect and do our best to navigate our careers. We can also be our own worst enemies. Arm yourself with positive strategies to navigate feelings of self-doubt.

Fear of failure

Underlying imposter syndrome is a fear of failure. You might think everyone wants to see you fail or that they will make fun of you if you fail. The truth is, everyone wants to see you succeed and "others" are probably too concerned with themselves to pay much attention.

If you do have people in your life who would like to see you fail, you need to stop giving them space in your mind. You're worth more than that! Everyone you bring into your circle should be invested in your success. Even people who don't think they have anything to contribute to your cause, will think about you when an opportunity arises or speak about you positively to others.

You're more than half way through this book, so hopefully you've identified some goals that excite you. You might also have felt a knee-jerk reaction that your goal is too big or far out to accomplish. That reaction is your ego trying to protect you from scary failure.

I define failure for myself—not as the tragic end to ambition, but as the failure to pursue the ambition in the first place. One failure I sometimes lament is that I didn't pursue psychiatric or mental health nursing early in my career, despite a strong desire to do so. Starting in undergrad, I felt that mental health nursing was up my alley. Fear of missing out, kept me saying "Yes" to opportunities that didn't align with my interests despite my gut telling me "No."

Imposter syndrome and fear of failure also resulted in my not pursuing an opportunity to write for an influential nursing journal. I was put in contact with the editor who was looking for an article by an "up and coming" nurse leader. Having only worked as a junior project manager for a few weeks, and with *only* an undergraduate degree, (still more formal education in academic writing than many experienced nurses had) I felt like I didn't have enough credentials - that I would be a fraud and my writing wouldn't be taken seriously.

Never mind that I had successfully organized a nursing conference of my making. Never mind that I had worked across several units—from medical-surgical to emergency to intensive care and recovery room. *Never mind* that I was the chair of the unit council and had influence at the hospital-wide nursing council. I still didn't consider myself a leader. I didn't have the title or master's degree that I thought I needed to be a *real* leader. And, I was afraid. So, despite the opportunity falling into my lap and the likelihood of being published in a nursing journal that I would have been tremendously proud of, I failed by shying away from the opportunity.

How do I manage fear now? I feel it but I focus on the *outcome* I expect to achieve. Once you understand the mechanics of how you can get to your outcome, you can put trust into the process. Your goals become achievable and you believe you can accomplish the things you set in motion.

What if that isn't enough? In that case, remind yourself of your successes. Reflect on all the big things you've been able to do in your life, and give yourself daily gold stars for small tasks you've accomplished. Celebrate!

Whenever there is something worth taking a risk for—something you desire, a shadow of doubt will come with it. It's inevitable. Overcoming the resistance is where success lies. Confidence and courage are the magic ingredients required.

EXERCISE: Imposter syndrome

1. Think of a time you experienced imposter syndrome. What was the trigger? What did it make you feel? What was your action?
2. Work through the five strategies for imposter syndrome outlined in this chapter.
3. Is fear holding you back from your career goals?
    a. Write down your fear and then write down your desired outcome.
    b. Write an example of a time you succeeded.
    c. When you feel your fear creeping in, remind yourself of your desired outcome and how you've had success in the past.

It's up to you to prioritize patient
numero uno - you! Not only is it up to
you, but it's a professional imperative.

MODULE 6

YOU: LIVING AUTHENTICALLY AND SELF-CARE!

"Self-care is giving the world the best of you, instead of what's left of you."
—Katie Reed

Taking care of yourself can be a source of pride, guilt or indifference. Know that you are worthy of putting yourself first. By the end of Module 6 you will understand the importance of showing up authentically, taking care of your body and mind, and putting yourself first. You will be able to identify authentic opportunities that align with your personal identity, be aware of your professional image and identity, and take control of your time, and mental, spiritual and physical health.

YOUR AUTHENTIC OPPORTUNITY

WHEN YOU BECOME A NURSE, your identity changes. This change can happen so gradually that you don't even notice. If you are not careful—at some point—you may no longer recognize your former self. In this module, we will take time to put *you* back into *your* career.

In nursing school, we're taught to care for our patients, then we work like we don't have our own physical bodies to care for. It wasn't until I became a Nurse Practitioner that I learned to prescribe self-care in the form of talk therapy, meditation, exercise, sleep and healthy nutrition. Even so, no one mentioned prescribing self-care to *myself*!

What if you put yourself on your patient list? "Ugh," you lament, "one more person to care for in my already overloaded schedule."

It's up to you to prioritize patient numero uno - *you*! Not only is it up to you, but it's a professional imperative. You have to fill your personal health and wellness cup so that you can pour into others and still have something left for yourself at the end of the day. That is the only way you can continue to support the patients and communities you serve. Authenticity and self-care are my secret weapons to long-term success.

Persistence Pays Off

Scribble, scribble, scribble. Erase, erase, erase. Scribble, scribble. Voilà! Perfection! After what was probably ten minutes, I had my masterpiece. It started with something like… roses are red, violets are blue, and then had an additional six lines of magic that only a six-year-old could come up with. Replete with spelling errors, I begged my parents to submit it to an address in the back of a magazine requesting submissions for poetry. We put it in an envelope, drew a stamp on the corner, and put it in the mailbox outside my front door. I eagerly waited for the phone call telling me that this was the best poem the publisher had ever read, and to offer me millions in publishing rights and a book deal. I love the confidence of six-year-old me!

My writing ambitions grew over time. I was never a *great* writer and received just average marks in English. That didn't stop a pull in my heart to write. After my first year of nursing school, I knew I wanted to write a book for nurses. I wrote this goal over and over again in my New Year's resolutions. It only took ten years to get started! As they say, the best time to plant a tree is ten years ago, the second best is now!

What would your six-year-old self, think of where you are today?

By now, you know I've embraced opportunities throughout my career—even when they weren't really what I was looking for. Over time, I learned to stop accepting every opportunity and avoiding growth challenges for fear of failure. You also know that I define failure not as getting an "F" on an exam, but as not taking steps toward your goals.

The popular phrase *fear of missing out* (FOMO) was the subconscious mind fork of my twenties that prevented me from directing my career in the direction I felt I wanted to pursue. I wouldn't grant myself the things that, deep down, I knew would make me authentically satisfied. Even my decision to pursue becoming an NP was directed by FOMO because I was scared to leave the clinical realm to pursue an MBA or nursing leadership program. In contrast, you can spot authentic ambition. It is relentless and stops at nothing.

An NP student, who I precepted, shared her story of getting into NP school. She hadn't applied herself in her undergraduate degree because she didn't anticipate wanting to do a master's degree afterward. As time went by, her colleagues suggested she should get her master's degree and go into leadership. Initially, she took their advice and applied (and got accepted) to a master's program on a part-time basis. But then, she realized that what she truly wanted was to become a Nurse Practitioner. She applied for the NP program three years in a row and was rejected each time. She was discouraged but determined.

With each rejection, she took the opportunity to meet with the course director, seeking advice on how she might be more likely to gain admission into the program. Each time, she was told that her undergraduate grades decreased her overall application score making admission unlikely. Despite facing multiple rejections, she persisted. She knew it was what she truly wanted. On her fourth try, she was finally admitted! And, I'm happy to say that she is now an NP with a career every bit as satisfying as she hoped.

STOP AND THINK

Are you are on a path aligned with your authentic self. Have you been accepting the status quo or saying yes to projects that steal your energy? Has fear of failure or of hearing "no" held you back? Make a promise to follow your dreams no matter the obstacle or number of years it takes to get there.

EXERCISE: Facing rejection

1. Was there a time you were rejected multiple times, but then succeeded?
2. Do you know someone who succeeded through persistence? What do you think rejection felt like? How do you think they ultimately felt when they were successful? What if they had stopped after the first no?
3. Think of a time you were offered an opportunity, but declined because you didn't think you were smart enough or experienced enough. Was there a time you had a goal, but put it on the back burner because you put the needs of others before your own?

YOUR PROFESSIONAL IMAGE

Introductions

Happy to make your acquaintance, my name is...hmm, how should I introduce myself? Mary, Nurse Mary, Nurse Practitioner Mary Ghazarian (my maiden name), Mrs. Wiseman (my married name), or just Nurse? Substitute my name for your name and repeat out loud. How does each of those feel to you? Did they sound too casual, too stuffy, or just right?

For the first two years of my career, I was either "Nurse" or Mary. When walking into a patient room my usual opening line was, "Hi, I'm Mary, I'll be your nurse today." After all, that's how I was taught to introduce myself in undergrad. Meanwhile, I had a colleague who would open with, "Hello, I'm Brandy, like the drink!"

While these aren't *bad* introductions, it turns out, these were the wrong way to go about building a professional career.

As nurses, we're often hesitant to give our last names, especially when working in high-risk areas like Emergency Departments. It's done for personal safety reasons but how can a patient send accolades to the patient relations department about the wonderful care you've provided when they don't know your last name? Instead, they will sing the praises of the doctor whose name and title they remember.

Consider this. Who would you feel more confident about piloting your plane— "Joe" or Captain Joseph Wright? I first learned about the importance of using your full name and title from author Suzanne Gordon. She asked me, "When you get on an aircraft and the flight attendant is going through the safety protocol, how do they introduce the pilot?" Likewise, patients, colleagues, and hiring managers will have a first impression about who you are based on your introduction.

I got positive feedback when I started sharing my full name. Patients started inquiring about the origins of my last name and this helped to build rapport and trust. My name started to be included in more "thank you" cards and I felt something different even within myself—increased confidence and ownership of my work.

Titles

I started working as a nurse before I got the passing result of my licensing exam but I remember the first time I was told, "You're the *nurse* now." Not being a nursing student or "nurse temp" as my badge read, my entire perspective changed. I felt responsible for my decisions. I was no longer under the protection of someone else's license. *I* was a nurse. *I* would care for *my* patients and their care was *my* responsibility—no longer the responsibility of a preceptor.

A new pathway awoke in my brain with the change in title from student to Registered Nurse. There was clarity and confidence instead of feeling like an imposter. The same thing happened when I went from Registered Nurse to Advanced Practice Nurse, and then from Advanced Practice Nurse to Nurse Practitioner. Not only did I feel different with each title change, but I was treated differently. When I was granted the title of Nurse Practitioner, my physician colleagues asked me to start calling them by their first names. I amassed a list of personal email addresses of specialists for direct contact instead of going through secretaries. Even though I was the same person, the new title brought a different perception from others.

While I may be respected by colleagues who are familiar with healthcare lingo, the title of Nurse Practitioner is still relatively unknown. When I introduce myself, I often get the response, "my mother/sister/cousin is a practical nurse too." And, in the executive health practice where I was first hired it was, "When will I see the doctor?" I educated people on my title almost every day, and I understand why. Before attending university,

I didn't know what nurses did and I didn't understand the different titles of RPN, RN, NP.

When someone asks what you do, how do you respond? Many nurses respond, "I'm *just* a nurse." If you have ever answered that way, consider this—is an astronaut "just an astronaut"?

Responding with your full title is a step up. "I'm a Registered Nurse," proudly takes ownership of your professional title. Yet, many people will still respond with, "My mother/sister/cousin is a nurse," and lump you in with a group, instead of recognizing you as an individual. I want you to be a member of a trusted professional group *and* a "nurse to know!"

Don't just *use* your title, *own* your title. One of the most useful exercises I've done to help people understand the significance of my title is to write an elevator pitch; a description of my job that I could give in the length of time it takes to get between floors on an elevator.

Picture this: The elevator doors open. You saunter in, spot your target (hospital CEO, politician, hiring manager, unassuming stranger), and after a few brief niceties, you start your speech. As a Nurse Practitioner, mine goes something like this:

> "A nurse practitioner is a registered nurse with advanced education and preparation who is licensed and authorized to diagnose, treat, and prescribe. This is similar to a doctor, but with the lens of nursing philosophy which considers the whole person. Nurse Practitioners deliver primary and specialty health care to all populations across the lifespan. Every quality study done to date supports nurse practitioners as high-quality, cost-effective health care providers."

You can develop an elevator speech that is specific to your unique area of specialty, interests, and accolades. I'm giving you permission to brag. You earned it!

Professional image

In my hospital, you could always distinguish the nursing leadership from the medical leadership. Physicians would wear the latest fashions, circulating throughout the unit in suits and dress shoes while most of the nurses wore wrinkled scrubs and sensible clogs with hairstyles that were well out of date.

We've come a long way since the days of starched white uniforms with caps and I don't think we should go back there, but I do think we still need to be mindful of the message we are conveying by our appearance. Eighty percent of communication is nonverbal. This includes our general appearance. We work really hard—really, really hard, but having a run-down appearance may not be doing us any favours in the increased recognition department.

In my tenure as a bedside nurse, I didn't wear a lick of makeup most days, because I didn't feel like my appearance mattered. I'd throw on a pair of hospital-issued baggy blue scrubs, throw my hair in a ponytail, lace my sneakers, and off I went to be a healthcare hero. It was simple and effective. On the rare professional education day, yoga pants and zipped hoodies were a common uniform. None of the nurses wore professional or business casual attire, unlike our physician colleagues who were never seen stepping into the hospital without a suit jacket.

Nurses often want to appear down-to-earth and approachable and this translates to our casual dress. Casual dress *is* actually appropriate in some settings, especially in areas like community health nursing. Be aware that it may not be sending the intended message when we are looking to advance our careers.

Looking the part of the role you hold, or aspire to have, helps others to envision you in that role. I'm not telling you to trade in your colourful scrubs for a grey suit. I'm not telling you to wear makeup or spend hundreds of dollars a year on manicures. All I'm saying is to be mindful of the non-verbal message you are sending. At a minimum, address body odours and basic hygiene, then the sky's the limit!

Online presence

Have you ever Googled your name? What is the first thing that comes up? Is it about you? Is it your personal social media account or professional LinkedIn account? Maybe you are a ghost online, completely unsearchable. Be mindful that the results of this search is also what any healthcare recruiter, human resource professional, or other colleague who is interested in learning more about you is likely seeing as well.

The internet gives you the opportunity to portray yourself in any light you choose. If you don't monitor what comes up in a Google search, you are leaving your fate to chance. Are you getting rejection letters because your Instagram account is showcasing your latest late-night escapade with a magnum-sized bottle of wine, instead of lessons from the latest educational course you took?

In an interview, Dr. Sonja Mitrevska Schwartzbach revealed that while she is an introvert, social media is a necessary part of marketing her work as an author. At the time of the writing of this book, she had over 50,000 followers on Instagram (find her on Instagram at @nursesonja). That level of popularity comes with great opportunity, and some disturbing realities, like people stealing her image and creating fake accounts. She largely relies on her followers to report fake accounts, and acknowledges that these accounts could lead to a negative portrayal of her but it's a reality on the internet that she can't control. What she *can* control is what she publishes and she does this with great care and consideration for what is appropriate, and not appropriate, to share on social media.

Some people shy away from the internet. They would rather be invisible. I recommend the opposite. Take control of what is in your control. While you may want to set your personal social media to private, take the opportunity to boost your professional image online. Think about the message your online presence sends. To what degree does sharing details of your personal life fit with that image?

Create or update your LinkedIn profile with your work, education, and volunteer experience. Consider creating a professional website—www.YourName.com—where you can create blog posts that showcase your expertise and invite others to connect with you. Virtually meeting other professionals who share your interests and who could help to move your career forward, is a real positive of our online world! Protect your online presence. It is as important to your career as the personal protective equipment you wear to shield yourself from infectious diseases.

Exercise: Your elevator pitch

1. Practice saying your name out loud in different ways with different combinations of your title, first name, and last name.
   a. Which of these do you prefer and why?
   b. What do you think each of these combinations says about you? Is someone nearby to give you an opinion? Ask them what they would prefer to hear if they were your patient or a physician colleague meeting you for the first time.
2. When someone asks what you do, how do you respond?
3. Write your elevator speech. This is a speech about yourself you can give in one minute. Think about why your story is important. What is your angle that is different from other nurses?

YOUR TIME

As I write this, I can see my neighbour in his front yard with a leaf blower getting debris off his lawn and onto the street (at least five feet away from his property). I'm waiting for him to pull out a tiny pair of scissors—about the size that comes in a suture kit— to snip the edges of his lawn and any stray blade of grass. He will repeat this tomorrow, and the following day and every other day, until a solid layer of snow covers his lawn. It is an immaculate lawn. I can't help but think that this daily ritual is actually an act of avoidance.

I too have spent a lot of time "procrasti-cleaning." In fact, I created a speaker series, an online course for overcoming imposter syndrome, *and* an online course on Nurse Practitioner entrepreneurship as I procrastinated from completing this book. I'm also guilty of misappropriating large amounts of time, of running on too few hours of sleep, of not taking vacation and of taking on a new role with a fancy title with no boundaries between work and life.

One thing we all have in common is time. What makes us different, is how we spend that time. Successful people spend their time pursuing what they need and want, not waiting for the fabled "right time" when stress magically disappears. When it comes to positive health habits, spending your time wisely is of utmost importance. We've already discussed "time," but time is so important that we're going to touch on it again. When time is spent on the wrong things, mental and physical health are going to fail.

Good habits go out the window when your cup is empty, and stress will build up like a steaming kettle until it screams and you can't ignore it anymore. Workouts, clean eating, home cooking, and sleep become a non-priority. Your mind and body are consumed by stress and something has to give.

"This?" you say, "This is all just temporary. Once this (insert stressful situation here) passes, I'll get back to my healthy habits and take care of myself." One week passes, then two—a month, a year. You may get past one hurdle only to have another appear. Stress becomes the new normal. And it shows.

Slight weight gain turns into 10 or 20-pounds. Or, maybe you have the opposite problem and can't keep weight on. What you thought would be one glass of wine with dinner, turns into a bottle. Relaxing in front of an episode of your favorite tv show becomes a binge session.

"If only I could escape and leave everything behind," is something I've heard expressed in my office from young adults, seniors, singles, parents, and CEOs alike. You may have had similar thoughts. In some cases, you may need to literally escape e.g., when in an abusive relationship with a spouse or employer. But, when you are in a cycle of self-abuse, physical escape is *not* the solution.

Have you been stuck in this cycle? Contemplating a change? Ruminating about your list of "I shoulds?" This is a cycle of self-abuse that looks like intimate partner violence, only it is with the ultimate of intimate partners—*yourself*!

I used to pile on work, then buy myself a fancy California red wine on my way home as consolation. I promised myself to start healthy habits, and to love myself more tomorrow. I drank half the bottle, ordered a pizza with my buzzed brain, and repeated the cycle the next day. I was waking up exhausted, skipping a morning workout or balanced breakfast in favour of running late to work and picking up a coffee and croissant along the way. I worked overtime when my boss asked me to. Then, I'd skip my evening workout with my trainer—choosing to pay their fee and not show up. This cycle was on repeat, until my wardrobe no longer fit. I invested in an all-black, loose and stretchy wardrobe. I stopped going to the hair salon and convinced myself I was no longer being superficial and instead was giving myself love and acceptance. It was a lie.

The gift of time

How did I break the cycle of violence against myself? I gave myself back one of the most valuable resources—time. First, the low-hanging fruit:

- I stopped going down the social media rabbit hole of scrolling. Check your screen time. You'll find hours! I switched to only using social media for wealth-building activities.
- I put some of my hard-earned money to work for me - investing $30 instead of buying a bottle of wine.
- I made boundaries. I stopped accepting work that wasn't moving the needle in my career and wasn't allowing me to enjoy the fruits of my labour.

Lastly, I took stock of the maintenance tasks in my life. I wrote a list that included doing dishes, laundry, vacuuming, changing the cat litter, grocery shopping, cooking, going to the gym, getting my nails and hair done, and visiting the dentist every three months. Like many women, most of the household maintenance tasks fell to me. I had to evaluate where I was wasting time and mental energy. I weighed these against financial cost.

Four hours of housework, taking out the garbage and recycling, an hour for grocery shopping, and a few more hours of food prep followed by doing dishes on the weekend could equal several hundred dollars in earning potential, if I spent that time doing other work.

If I enjoyed doing household tasks and they brought me joy—I sometimes relish a good closet-organizing afternoon—then the money wouldn't matter. Instead, I often resented these tasks. I would stare at my husband sitting on the couch and feel angry that he was able to relax while my hamster-wheel-mind was thinking about all the chores to be done.

Once I saw (in writing) where I felt I was wasting my time, I was able to justify outsourcing many of the maintenance tasks. I hired a cleaner and invested in an organic meal prep delivery service for breakfast, lunch, and dinner six days a week.

I felt a lot of resistance to paying for these services; they were for "rich people" or "lazy people." However, my husband had grown up with a nanny and housekeeper, and once I was relieved of the stress associated with the tasks I delegated, I regretted not hiring help sooner.

In our gym business, we pay for a bookkeeper, accountant, manager, cleaner, social media team, and so on. Having staff help means the gym operates, more or less, on autopilot so I can work as a Nurse Practitioner. I had to make the same investments in my personal life where possible.

Sometimes you just have to pay the money for the right solutions. For you, it might not be hiring a cleaner. It could be hiring a repair person to fix the dishwasher or laundry machine. It could also be taking a course to learn low-cost healthy cooking or time management.

I'm not saying to go into debt to hire a housekeeper, but figure out what activities you can eliminate or outsource. Ask for help. Instead of burying yourself in work, pursue activities that fill your soul and recharge your energy. Set boundaries and protect your time as your most valuable asset.

Using time wisely

Once you rediscover having time in your day, it's important not to squander it. Journaling, meditation, playing with your kid or visiting friends, travel, and gardening are things that can give you joy and a renewed sense of purpose.

And speaking of purpose, pursue goals that energize you. Once you identify a goal, find the path of least resistance and invest in it. That might mean paying a coach, or finding a mentor. You could also invest in a course where the outcome is predetermined, saving you more time and energy:

- Take X course, get X designation, and work in X field or
- Work with X coach, overcome X barriers, and grow personally, professionally, and financially.

STOP AND THINK

If you feel you have unmet needs, use your journal to work it through. What do you really need to accomplish self-care and breathing space in your life? Is it just an hour at the gym? Is it taking up a creative pursuit? Is it a half-day, a week, a month, or a one-year sabbatical? What answer did you land on and why? (Really why—the honest why?) Identify one actionable step you can take. Do you need to tell your boss? Your spouse? Find a gym with a daycare space?

Can't answer these on your own? Find a counselor to help you get over a mental block.

Exercise: The time is now

1. What would you do with more time?
2. What is one actionable step you can take to make it possible?
3. Who do you need to recruit to help?

YOUR MENTAL AND SPIRITUAL HEALTH

Our brains are simple things. They love familiar patterns that allow them to run on autopilot and conserve energy. If your autopilot is running a pattern of negativity, anxiety or despair—no amount of time or money will solve your problems or make you happy. Negative programming needs to change to bring about the outcomes you are looking for.

What does a typical negative pattern look like? Cognitive behavioral therapy tells us the pattern is: *thoughts* lead to *feelings* that lead to *actions*. For example, you think studying for an exam is hard (thought), you feel dread (feeling) so, you procrastinate (action). This forms a repeating pattern until you replace it with a new pattern; better thoughts leading to better feelings and actions.

Negative thoughts, feelings and behaviours

A patient walked into my office in extreme distress. Their voice was shaky. They could barely look up from their trembling hands. They weren't sleeping. They weren't eating. They confided that they were worried about their spouse's demanding family coming to stay with them over the summer. They were even more worried about what their spouse would think if they told them how they felt.

Little did this person know that I had received a desperate call from their spouse that same morning. Out-of-character changes, like mistakes while cooking told the spouse that something was wrong. I was charged with getting to the bottom of it. In the end, both partners shared similar fears. At a bit of a loss for how best to help them, I referred the couple to counseling.

A few weeks later, my patient returned grinning from ear to ear. I thought perhaps their extended family had decided not to stay with them after all. Instead, they revealed the secret to their newfound happiness.

And, I am sharing this secret with you, because compelling secrets are meant to be shared.

Their therapist had advised that staying quiet and not communicating was the root cause of their anxiety. If the couple discussed what was on their minds, their anxiety would all but disappear— and it did!

Anxiety is caused when we think negative thoughts about a future that has not even come to pass. When we make negative assumptions about how things *might* be if we take an uncomfortable action, then we stop ourselves from expressing our true selves. Cognitive dissonance and discomfort arise. Until we change our thought patterns or act in line with our true desires, our anxiety is perpetuated.

Changing your patterns

The first step in change is awareness. Become aware of your thoughts by keeping a "thought log" including *thoughts*, *feelings*, and *actions*. At first, you'll find you have a lot of different thoughts. Then, within a few days, you'll notice that thoughts repeat themselves, especially the pesky negative ones that tell you your teeth aren't quite as white as you'd like them to be, or you really should get rid of all of your old underwear.

You'll know you're experiencing a negative thought when you feel a bit more (or a lot more) down than you would like. You might feel irritated or angry. Sometimes we notice a feeling first. If this is you, backtrack and ask yourself what thought brought on the feeling?

Sometimes, we only notice negativity after we've already taken the action—after drinking that third glass of wine for example. Again, backtrack to the feeling and thought. You were feeling low and thought the third glass of wine would be the thing to bring up your mood.

When recording your thoughts, feelings and actions, give yourself some grace. Don't judge yourself. Be impartial as possible.

After a week, consider which thoughts were most distressing and which thoughts formed a repeating pattern. Start here. One by one, rewrite a more ideal thought pattern to replace it. When the thoughts are especially distressing— "I *hate* my life and everyone in it,"—changing it to "I *love* my life and everyone in it" will not feel genuine. You may even feel worse. Instead, write down a more neutral thought, "I *have* a life and people in it." The next time you notice the pattern repeating, replace it with your new improved thought. Once you get comfortable with this the neutral thought, you can move towards something more positive. Start inviting new, more positive, patterns into your brain.

Sometimes the problem is bigger than your outlook. It's important you access the health resources you need—whether that is a local helpline, your primary care provider, therapist, or the emergency department. It might be a medical or psychosocial issue rather than a false belief that is holding you hostage. It is never too late to seek out help.

Compassion fatigue and burnout

At my lowest point, while working as an ICU nurse, there were many times when I felt I couldn't do even one more shift. My heart wasn't in it. I couldn't see one more person on futile life support. I couldn't change the intravenous lines of one more IV pump tree of vasopressors and anesthetics. I couldn't suction any more gunked-up endotracheal tubes. I couldn't stand the beeping of the monitors when an electrocardiogram sticker came loose. I came close to the end of my rope in nursing, but I didn't tell anyone. I was afraid of looking weak and felt burdened by the guilt of having my physical health, when my patients had it so much worse than me.

I had recurring dreams of extremely unfortunate events that could only take place in nursing. These were scenarios that had never even occurred in my real life, but which left me feeling highly anxious. I dreamt I forgot a patient all day, leaving them without assistance. I would have follow-up dreams too, of a nurse manager sitting me down and telling me about imaginary patients who passed away because of my negligence. I started to get palpitations just by stepping onto the unit.

- Do you walk onto your unit and immediately recall the time you almost gave the wrong dose of insulin to the patient in room 104, bed B?
- Do you occasionally call in sick because you dread the gossip of your co-workers?
- Do you find yourself staying silent, even though you want to tell your manager how unhappy you are with staffing ratios?
- Maybe you've had enough of talking about tough clients over dinner, but have forgotten what polite dinner conversation feels like!

If any of these resonate with you, you might be experiencing compassion fatigue or burnout. Don't hold these recurring distressing thoughts to yourself for fear of judgment. Let them out!

Write them in a journal or share them with your dog on a morning walk. Then, talk to a counselor, a supportive colleague, your manager, the CEO of the hospital, your union rep, a newspaper columnist…tell the world. Whatever you do, don't grip too tightly on your discomfort, or you will get to keep it.

I describe my initial entanglements with burnout and compassion fatigue as a complete shutdown of my personal life and basic emotions—happiness and sadness. Devoid of emotion, I felt like a high-functioning robot.

I shut off for so long that I forgot how to experience the world outside of 12-hour shifts. I developed thick skin, never crying for my patients or with their families. I never said no to a task. I never said no to a learning opportunity or lateral move from department to department. In the first two years of my nursing career, I never took a vacation. I went from opportunity to opportunity eventually landing as a nurse in multiple Intensive Care Units (ICUs).

I hustled while my adrenal glands worked overtime.

I drank mimosas at 7 am after night shifts with colleagues, as we joked that the alcohol would help us sleep through the day. Then, I downed a few large black coffees on the next shift to get me through.

I remember feeling emotionally dead in moments that should have brought joy, like a birthday dinner surrounded by friends in a posh downtown restaurant. "Bring on the champagne," I thought, "I need to feel *something*." I knew my brain was not going to be disinhibited enough to feel happy until I downed half a bottle!

One warm summer night at a cottage in Muskoka, Ontario, I watched the water sparkling from the light of the moon. It was a beautiful, serene moment in nature. The rhythmic sound of waves lapping against the wooden dock along with the occasional loon call kept me company. I knew I should be feeling peace and gratitude. I *wanted* to feel those things. Instead, I felt nothing. I could not even fake a smile.

When you live under duress, with caffeine and alcohol as your main fuel sources, your hormones change to favour stress hormones. My hormonal pathways had been geared up for stress for so long that I couldn't switch my brain chemistry, even in a quiet moment.

Serotonin! Where was my serotonin?

I got a lot of compliments. "You're so patient," my colleagues would say. From my manager, "You're so resilient." From friends and family, "You're so smart and successful! I'm so glad I can always come to you for advice." Ah, there were my small serotonin boosts; compliments.

Despite the accolades, I went for long periods of time without feeling happy. My patience and resilience may have started out as strengths, but I had retreated into them. Underlying my newly acquired flat affect, my primary emotions were feeling anxious and annoyed. I was a nurse. I was also,

- Burnt out.
- On the verge of alcohol addiction.
- Experiencing compassion fatigue.

Compassion fatigue is brought on by the negative emotions that come with working with people in distress. This fatigue started while working in the ICU. I felt like I was participating in the daily demise of human guinea pigs. Heroic efforts were made to save people from death at all costs, including their dignity. Anyone who has worked in a modern ICU will tell you that there are patients who are barely recognizable as humans; cannulated in nearly every orifice. Where no orifice naturally exists, new ones will be created. No part of the body is sacred—internal or external. The nuisance of bodily function is managed strategically. Neurosurgical or brain-injured patients were arguably the worst. I participated in (what would be considered torture in any other setting) waking patients every 15 minutes to check and make sure they were alive and in the same condition as they were the previous hour.

What could make you go a day without eating, peeing, or sitting down? What could be so important to make you forget your own basic needs? The first things that come to mind are being in a war zone or natural disaster. Add bedside nursing to the list. At any moment I had to be prepared for the unpredictable.

Pop culture paints a picture of nurses as hand-holders. In reality, there was little time for pleasantries or comforting hand-holding in the ICU. There were many times I was pulled away from a conversation with a person waiting for a transplant of some vital organ. If they survived, weeks and months of poking and prodding ahead of them. So many times, I had to walk away from people who were looking for some hope and humanity. I listened quietly, nodding along as long as I could, but usually limited to only a few minutes. I would have to get on to my next task or sacrifice a bathroom break. My solution was often to recommend a psychiatry or spiritual care consult to ensure human connection didn't get sacrificed.

I also dealt with uncertainty and guilt. There were countless times I wondered if I made the right decision. Should I have bothered the resident doctor one more time, or even gone above the resident to their attending? Should I have made one more round of the unit? And so on.

I will never forget the passing of a patient who went into cardiac arrest twice in one evening but had been deemed stable. Following the second code blue, his circulation returned through heroic efforts, leaving blood and bodily fluids in the wake of Advanced Cardiac Life Support. Another nurse and I cleaned him up. We changed the bedsheets and allowed the family in to see him. He looked quiet and comfortable, though not conscious. Rather than subjecting the family to another night in the waiting room, we reassured them their loved one was stable. They left. Fifteen minutes later, his heart stopped. I felt extreme guilt for sending his family away, but how were we to know?

An emergency room colleague came back to work after sustaining a workplace injury. He puttered about, relegated to an area where most of the patients were waiting to be admitted and moved up to a unit. My colleague wasn't ready for more acute cases—the ambulance bay, where patients with heart attacks and strokes would be rolled directly in. We all expected to pick up the slack since he had been away for a while. From 7 am to 10 am I watched as my colleague picked up and then put down charts while slowly wandering in and out of patient rooms. To the untrained eye, it looked like he was doing his job but a few hours into the shift, it was obvious there was no real action being taken. Orders on the charts weren't signed off and I could see my colleague struggling to stay awake.

I wish I could say it was me who took notice, but I was a new nurse who assumed everyone who came to work was a consummate professional. I didn't suspect anything. Instead, someone else spoke to the charge nurse who took our inebriated colleague aside. It turned out the returning nurse was high on the painkillers he was taking to treat pain. It was a real-life cautionary tale of nurses who lose their licenses due to patient endangerment and neglect. I don't know what happened next, but I never saw the nurse again. This was a case of someone with a workplace injury who returned to work too soon. I saw how easy it was to become a statistic.

Maybe you don't work in an ICU or emergency department and never plan to. Even as a Primary Health Care NP, I am still vulnerable to compassion fatigue.

The timing of returning to school to become an NP coincided with a major shift in my self-care. I got a personal trainer and meal-prepped religiously for optimal health. I quit alcohol. I decreased caffeine. I dropped twenty pounds!

In that blissful time, I regained my confidence and built a strong personal connection with my (now) husband. I made it through the NP program and Master's degree in good health. But, after starting my first full-time NP position, perfectionism and the tendency to please others instead of putting my needs first, re-emerged stronger than ever. With my increased responsibilities and prestige, came pressure to perform.

Outside of work, I was subconsciously assessing everyone's health. Even on the day of my wedding, I was so preoccupied with my husband's sore back that I couldn't enjoy standing at the wedding altar for our vows, worried about his potential discomfort from the prolonged standing. I didn't even consider that the glistening sweat on his forehead might have been from nerves, instead I assumed it was from pain. At one of the most important moments of my life, I was worried for my husband and annoyed at our luck that his back would be injured the week of our wedding.

Over three years I gained back more weight than I'd previously lost. I went from feeling confident and energized, to miserable and chronically tired. The weight didn't actually bother me, I learned to love my new body and maintain a healthy body image for the first time in my life. Unfortunately, the inability to keep up my three times per week weight training, binging carbs in secret, and indulging in wine were not in line with my message as an Executive Health NP who was preaching prevention and healthy lifestyle.

There are small and more obvious signs of compassion fatigue and burnout. Are you forgetting to cross your t's and dot the i's? Have you made "rookie" mistakes? Maybe you're doing more "chair nursing" than you should be. Instead of getting up to answer a call bell, you're wheeling yourself around the nursing station or ducking into a supply closet to make yourself scarce. Instead of advocating, you are passing the responsibility off to someone else, hoping for the best. It's important to recognize these red flags.

Preventing compassion fatigue and burnout

If you're in primary health care or health coaching, ask yourself, "Am I investing more of myself in managing this person's healthcare than they are?" If yes, take a step back.

If you're in a hospital, long-term care, or community setting, ask yourself, "Am I depriving myself of my basic human needs?" If yes, take a break.

Participate in regular debriefing with a trusted colleague or counselor. Make time for self-care by making sure you're taking vacation, using mental wellness and sick days as well as scheduling in healthy activities like exercise, meditation, and journaling. Staffing is not *your* problem unless you are a manager or director, in which case encourage your bedside staff to take well-earned time off.

Post-traumatic growth

How do you come back from compassion fatigue or burnout? How about recovering from abusive patients, a medical error, or a legal accusation? What about coping with the realities of inequitable or rationed care?

The saying goes—"in life only two things can be guaranteed: death and taxes." In nursing, I think the saying would be that witnessing death and medical errors are the only guarantee. Since two pandemics have taken place during my career, I'm also tempted to add pandemics to the list. The point is, that nurses witness or experience significant trauma in their careers.

Post-traumatic growth can be facilitated through education, emotional regulation, disclosure, narrative development, and service. Growth takes place through appreciation of life, personal strength, recognizing new possibilities, having relationships with others, and spiritual change. A dedicated nurse named Alex[12] suffered a severe injury while caring for a patient with a history of violence. The incident left Alex physically and emotionally traumatized, causing them to question their ability to continue in nursing. Through extensive therapy, support from loved ones, and their own resilience, Alex embarked on a remarkable journey of post-traumatic growth. They found solace in advocacy work, raising awareness about workplace safety and spearheading initiatives to provide better protection and training for healthcare workers, turning their own painful experience into a catalyst for positive change.

In the aftermath of a medical error resulting in post-traumatic stress, you may choose to leave your unit because of shame or an inability to move past the event. With post-traumatic *growth*, you seek opportunities to prevent a similar event from happening to someone else— through research, education, quality improvement, or product redesign or invention. Same nurse, same error—two possible outcomes.

Some people naturally veer toward growth. Others will need the help of a psychologist and/or medication. If you've experienced a traumatic event and the memory is haunting you, work with your HR department, manager, and personal healthcare team (including your primary care provider) to move towards growth.

Appreciation of life

What are the odds of you being here, at this moment in time in history? When I get into a negative spiral, I like to remember how lucky I am to even be alive. A "gratefulness log" can help lift you from a fog of despair. Write down five things you are grateful for. They can be things that have

---

12 *Name changed for confidentiality

happened, things that you see in your immediate vicinity, or things that haven't happened that you imagine will be in your future. Take this a step further by letting others know you appreciate them. For example, when I end an interaction with a patient, I don't just end the conversation with "take care," I say "pleasure meeting you today." And, I mean it.

Personal strength

18 months into the COVID-19 pandemic I encountered an old colleague. We started nursing the same year as part of the Nursing Resource Team. She ultimately found her spot in the Emergency Department. I asked her how she was, imagining that working in the ER during a pandemic must have been extremely difficult. She told me a lot of nurses left during the pandemic, but she felt it wasn't that bad—the patient volume was actually down as people avoided the hospitals for fear of getting sick. How was she able to stick it out? Resilience.

Having started her career by floating floor-to-floor on a daily basis, she had developed the ability to adapt in the face of uncertainty. For every shift she didn't know who she would be working with, or the type of ailments she would be dealing with. Instead, each morning she would retrieve a message telling her, "Today you will be on unit X." It wasn't until the hour before her shift started that she would know it would be a cardiology day...unless she got to work and was floated to another floor due to some external factor. Years of expecting the unexpected helped her during the pandemic, while others left the profession altogether. We can all build resilience by exposing ourselves to unfamiliar situations, continuing to learn new skills on a regular basis.

Spiritual health

Over the course of my career, I have witnessed death and miracles. I will never forget the young woman who wheeled herself back into my unit after spending several months unconscious due to a failed suicide attempt. For months she had no voluntary movement. The team thought she was destined for a life in a hospital bed. Many felt the situation was futile, but her brain stem was working so we continued to provide care. Eventually, she opened her eyes, then made sounds and words, then she moved her limbs. She had no memory of her time in the ICU, or the incident that landed her there, but she was happy to be alive. We were thrilled to see this miraculous human come back from the brink.

If there is any profession that comes close to witnessing all stages of life, it's nursing. It is hard to work in extremes and not contemplate your own mortality, spirituality, and the afterlife. Spirituality can mean a lot of things: your religion, your beliefs, your practices. My childhood was spent in the cult of the Worldwide Church of God, then in the Baptist church. In my teens and early twenties, I didn't attend any church. In my thirties, I married into a Jewish family. While religion in my life has been fluid, the concept of spirituality has stayed with me. The idea that there is something greater than myself at work, keeps me humble and prevents my ego from getting too big or too hurt.

Wherever you are in your beliefs, I encourage you to get yourself to the spiritual gym. Self-care isn't just about eating more green vegetables and getting in more exercise. It's also taking time to appreciate things in the moment. Don't wait until the end of your life, to reflect on all you've done. Personal reflection combined with assessing where you are in the present, will give you the mental strength to go forward.

Strengthen your spirit by practicing gratitude, positive affirmations, and mindfulness.

Gratitude allows us to recognize the good in our lives. You can practice gratitude through small rituals; like saying grace at meals or by noting things you're grateful for in a journal. Positive affirmations help bring your mindset back to the positive. For example, "All I need is within me right now." Mindfulness is the practice of being in the present rather than focusing on the past or future. My favourite mindfulness activity is to savour a sip of wine or bite of chocolate as if it's the first time I'm tasting it—paying special attention to the smell, flavor, and texture.

The take-away

I want you to know it's ok to not be ok but, I encourage you to seek help *before* you think you need it. Practice mental health wellness in the good times, so that you will have resilience when things become challenging. Embrace your discomfort—understanding its purpose in identifying what is out of sync with your expectations and for reminding you that you are human. Then, move forward. Know that life is a series of lessons. Be curious. Do not rush the future. Take the time to reflect on your experiences.

Exercise: Take a mental health inventory

1. How have you been feeling lately? Rate your mental and spiritual health on a scale of 0-10. If it is not a 10/10, what would it take to move that number in a positive direction by even one point?
2. It is never too soon to find resources to support your mental health. If you have the financial means or benefit coverage, consider taking even one session with a therapist to learn how therapy may help you.
3. Do an internet search for local mental health resources. Consider finding a local place of worship. Check out apps that may help you form healthy mindfulness habits.
4. Use positive affirmations: Write down a positive phrase that you will see and repeat to yourself throughout your day.

YOUR PHYSICAL HEALTH

"Remember to drink water and get some sun. We are basically houseplants with more complicated emotions."

—Unknown

We're taught to care for our patients, then we work like we don't have our own physical bodies to look after. What if you put yourself on your patient list? "Ugh," you lament, "one more person to care for in my already overloaded schedule."

It's up to you to prioritize patient numero uno - you! Not only is it up to you, but it's a professional imperative. You *have* to put on your oxygen mask first, so you can survive to support the patients and communities you serve.

We all need healthy movement, nutrition, sleep, and a positive environment to be highly functional nurses. Let's explore these further.

Injury prevention

He stood at the foot of the bed and stared downward. Unblinking eyes welled with tears. "Her feet," he muttered as I stood by his side, "swimmer's feet." They were covered in blankets, so I could only imagine what swimmer's feet looked like. Webbed like a duck? Fins perhaps? He continued, "My daughter's an Olympian you know." I didn't. I had just started a shift in the neuro step-down unit and hadn't received that bit of information in the report. I knew that a severed spinal cord meant she would never use those feet again. The perfect wriggling ten toes her father counted on the day of her birth, and the two feet that kicked expertly all the way to the winners' podium—were now still.

As we stood there silently, my thoughts turned to my "nurse's feet." For three years my feet had carried me countless miles through city streets, onto the subway, through the hospital doors, up and down the corridors of the units, and back home again.

I thanked my feet.

Having taken my feet for granted until this point, I started to think about a future without them. Without my nurse's feet, how would I still be a nurse?

I had never thought far ahead in my career or considered that disability could be a part of my future. The "what ifs" started flowing. *What if* I lose my mobility? *What if* I couldn't run around the unit from call bell to call bell? *What if* I couldn't crouch, lunge, squat, and otherwise maneuver myself to assist my patients? *What if* I couldn't be a bedside nurse? Did I want to be one forever? Despite being worthy of a gold medal for (what often felt like) completing the most steps on a nursing unit in one shift, there was no extra recognition for the job my feet did.

Protect your back, your knees, your shoulders, and all your other body parts from injury, and your legs from varicose veins. Always insist on using a lifting device, using proper body mechanics, and having assistance for transfers. Arguably, nurses are seen as disposable, so injuries are often overlooked for more pressing organizational issues. Take steps to prevent a career-ending injury and look forward to a pain-free retirement.

Movement

With charting requirements getting longer and more work moving online, we spend more hours sitting than ever before.

Throughout my career, moving from department to department also meant I was slowly spending less time walking. I would get more than 15,000 steps a day on a medical/surgical unit. In the ICU, ten steps to the patient and back to my desk, a few times an hour was often all that was required. With less physical activity my scrubs gradually became too tight. I imagine this was the fate of many of my colleagues who suffered from preventable health issues despite having the education to know better.

I tried to get into running. I bought a fancy high-tech running watch to track my distance, pace, and heart rate for outdoor runs, and a treadmill for rainy or cold days. I started off strong— for a week or two. Then the watch found its way to a junk drawer and my treadmill became a clothes-drying rack.

I needed an intervention. My friend owned a personal training studio and invited me to join. I made a goal to get below 20% body fat. Within six months I had accomplished my goal by training with a personal trainer 3 times a week and recording my food intake. I loved lifting weights. It was very challenging the first three months, but finally my body got the memo that it needed to lift heavy things and handle increased cardiovascular work. I started to look forward to making new goals for the number of chin-ups I could do, or the weight in my bench press.

My scrubs were loose again. I was feeling confident and energetic. I started wearing makeup to work. I smiled more. I was more positive. I felt successful instead of stuck.

What was the difference between running and weightlifting? I hated running and I enjoyed weightlifting. I had a natural disdain for one and an affinity for the other. Science tells us that when we pursue activities we hate, it raises our cortisol—the stress hormone. When we do things we enjoy, we raise our dopamine—the happy hormone. Guess which one you're more likely to continue to return to time and time again? That's right! The one you enjoy! So, pick a type of physical activity you enjoy and stop guilting yourself into learning to love the things you don't. Life is too short for that.

Nutrition

I spent much of my young adulthood as a vegetarian because I didn't like the thought of eating animals. At the age of 15, I told my mother, "I won't eat anything with eyes." Eggs were ok in my books, but no fish, poultry, pork, or beef for me. At the time, there were few resources on vegetarianism and few plant-based meat substitutes. I became a junk food vegetarian—eating a lot of bread and cookies and not so many vegetables. I'm pretty sure I stunted my growth, as I now stand at least a head shorter than my siblings.

By the time I turned 21, my body was craving meat. Likely low on iron and vitamin B12, I started to sneak meat—usually in the form of a few cold cuts on visits to my mother's house. Then, on a solo trip to Las Vegas, I ordered steak frites at a fancy restaurant. By the time I returned home, it was official. I was no longer vegetarian.

Unfortunately, having spent my teens not eating meat, I didn't know how to cook it. Instead of taking a course or opening a cookbook, I started ordering in. I never brought lunch to work and I always stopped at a coffee shop for a morning donut. For lunch and dinner, I went to the hospital food court to pick up whatever looked good. As the years went by and my metabolism slowed, my body made it clear that this strategy was also not going to work.

Once again it was my personal trainer friend (now husband) Jonathan, to the rescue. The guidelines were simple. "The best diet," he said, "is the one that you can stick to." Then he outlined the plan. Four meals a day. Each meal was to have a serving of protein, a cup of vegetables, and a healthy carb like oats. Fruits were for after workouts along with a protein source to replenish what I'd used up. Dark chocolate in the evening with a glass of wine if I wanted. And, one day a week, I could throw the rules out the window.

Following these guidelines along with regular workouts, got me into the best shape of my life. I felt more energy than even in my teens. Now, anytime I'm feeling low energy I can look back at my diet habits and see that usually, I've been too low on protein and vegetables. Within two weeks of going back to healthy habits, my energy will rebound.

The right nutrition for me, is not necessarily the right nutrition for you. So many factors come into play including ancestry and preferences but, I do believe a plant-based diet with adequate protein is superior to a diet high in processed foods. Also, the culture of starvation dieting needs to go. Even with weight loss efforts, you need enough calories for your brain and hormones to function well. Better to eat more of the right foods than no food at all. Consider seeing a dietician for personalized advice.

Sleep

Shift work, working multiple jobs, having a baby, being a caregiver, studying for exams—at some point we all experience sleep deprivation. In the short-term, we cope with fatigue, some lack of coordination, and poor memory that can be equivalent to the effect of having three alcoholic beverages. In the long-term, lack of sleep increases our stress hormones and puts other hormones out of whack, leading to chronic illness. For example, the risk of heart disease increases the longer a nurse works shift work.[13] After just 72 hours, sleep deprivation can lead to hallucinations and cognitive deficits. Extreme circumstances can lead to death.

It is easy to see that sleep is a vital part of our everyday lives. We each need between 7-9 hours of sleep a night so, it's important to prioritize downtime and take care of *you*. When you're rested and recharged, you can accomplish more and support others better. It's not selfish because you'll have more of yourself to give.

I used to cope with night shifts by napping on my break. It turns out that restorative napping strategy is well-documented in the literature, however many workplaces are against the idea of catching a few zzz's while on shift.[14] Nevertheless, if another nurse is covering your patients, and you are accessible in case of emergency, napping can be an effective strategy to prevent sleep deprivation. It is the norm in many

---

13 Vetter et al. 2016
14 Mcmillan, D & Fallis, W. (2011). Benefits of napping on night shifts. *Nursing Times* [online]; 107: 44, 12-13.

male-dominated professions such as police and fire, and the evidence tells us this should be seen as a safety measure rather than a safety hazard!

If your life circumstances are such that there is no time for sleep, take micro naps when possible and consider enlisting some help. If you are experiencing difficulty falling asleep and/or staying asleep use the checklist below to improve your sleep and gain energy!

Top tips for healthy sleep:[15]

1. *Create a comfortable sleep environment.* Block out light, get the room temperature just right, and minimize noise.

2. *Use the bedroom for one of two things: sleep or sex.* Avoid making the bedroom your home office.

3. *Create a relaxing wind-down routine.* Take a bath, meditate, or journal.

4. *Have a snack.* Choose foods high in tryptophan like cheese, turkey, or peanut butter, and pair them with a carbohydrate like an apple or toast. Avoid high-sugar foods or heavy meals before bed.

5. *Get physical!* Be active during the day aiming for 30 minutes of physical activity. Avoid exercising too close to bedtime.

6. *Wake up at the same time every day.* Waking at the same time in the morning will ensure you are tired at the same time every night, helping to regulate your sleep and wake hormones. What if you work shift work? Use natural light or artificial light with 10,000 lux to reset your internal clock when you wake up.

7. *Sleep only when sleepy.* If you get into bed and feel wide awake, get up and do something relaxing for 20 minutes rather than lying awake in bed. Return to bed when you are sleepy.

8. *Keep a journal beside your bed.* Write down your thoughts and to-do list before bed. Use the journal if you wake through the night

---

[15] https://www.uptodate.com/contents/image/print?imageKey=SLEEP%2F122804

and find it difficult to fall back to sleep due to worry or recurring thoughts.

9. *Avoid caffeine, nicotine, and alcohol.* Caffeine and nicotine are stimulants. Avoid them in the afternoon and evening. Alcohol is a depressant and helps you feel sleepy, but contributes to poor-quality sleep and sleep apnea.

10. *Turn off your phone, tablet, computer, and television.* Bright blue light from technology delays the production of the sleep hormone melatonin and sleep onset. If you are tempted to look at text messages or social media through the night, turn off your tech and leave it outside of the bedroom.

11. *Skip the nap.* If you have trouble falling asleep it might be because you caught up on your sleep in the afternoon. Avoid naps to reset your sleep cycle.

12. *Use a sleep diary to chart your progress.* Tracking your habits and making small changes over time will lead to success. Track your progress to stay motivated

Tried all of the above and still not getting a good night's sleep? Cognitive behavioural therapy for insomnia (CBT-I) is an evidenced-based talk therapy treatment. On the other hand, if you are sleeping eight hours a night and are still tired, or if you snore, make an appointment with your primary care provider to ask about a sleep study to rule out underlying causes of unrefreshing sleep like sleep apnea.

Environment

I once worked with a nurse from Vancouver, British Columbia. When she joined the Cardiovascular Surgery Intensive Care Unit she was experienced in the specialty. I asked her how she liked Toronto compared to back home. "Everything is the same," she replied, "but also completely different." Despite the same protocols, patient population, and acuity she was ten times as stressed. A few months later she was feeling ready to leave nursing altogether but instead of hanging up her stethoscope, she returned to the west coast. She returned to her old unit and found happiness again. When I asked her what changed she replied, "The environment."

In Toronto, none of her coworkers took lunch breaks outside together. Instead, they sat quietly and socially distanced (before social distancing was a public health recommendation) in front of the blue light of the television playing a 24-hour news station. Instead of easy day trips into the wilderness or going to the beach with friends on days off, she was surrounded by a bustling noisy city polluted with smog.

While we can't all live by the ocean, we *can* recognize that our work culture and the environments we spend our time in impact our physical health. How many Juliet balconies let fresh air and the sounds of the birds in at your workplace? How many weeks or months pass where you don't feel sunlight on your face because it's winter or you're working night shifts? How often do you step into your workplace and immediately feel your heart rate and blood pressure rise?

Working indoors is the modern epidemic. Believe it or not, Chronic Obstructive Pulmonary Disorder (COPD) occurs in non-smoking office workers in a similar incidence as in smokers.[16] This tells us that indoor air can be worse than outdoor air. The easy transmission of COVID-19 in poorly ventilated areas also highlighted the importance of good indoor air quality.

You don't need to move across the country to find a better environment. Instead, scan for simple improvements that you can make. Increase your time spent outdoors in the fresh air and natural sunlight. If you live in a city, make a point to visit green space on a regular basis. Get sun—even in winter. Do a deep clean and organization of your home.

---

16 Syamlal et al. 2021

Exercise: Taking care of YOU

1. Movement: Write down three activities you enjoy, that get your heart rate up. Schedule them into your week

2. Nutrition: Record your diet from the last 24-hours.
    - Are you getting adequate protein, fruits, vegetables, and healthy fats?
    - Are you drinking enough water?
    - Are you dining out more than you would like?
    - Are you overindulging in caffeine, surgery beverages, fast food, or alcohol?
    - Identify nutritional change to work on for the next week. Consider speaking with a nutritionist for professional advice.

3. Sleep: Track your sleep for one week, then review the sleep hygiene tips and adopt one change to improve your sleep habits.

4. Environment: What one change can you make today to increase your happiness?

YOUR PERSONAL IDENTITY

My maiden name is Ghazarian (pronounced Guh-zair-ee-uhn). Growing up with a unique last name, compared to a sea of Smiths and Johnsons, was both a blessing and a curse. My name has been simplified by many to be Mary 'G.' While I resented having a *different* last name growing up, as an adult I've grown to appreciate it. A unique name is a great conversation starter and a surefire way to be remembered.

The origin of my name is Armenian. My father and his family emigrated to Canada to escape genocide. They brought delicious food, traditions, and the last name. On the other hand, my mother is a European Canadian going back several generations. I think most would agree I look Caucasian, but I identify as having a mixed heritage, as I never felt quite *as white as* my peers in the small suburb where I grew up.

When I married, I had a difficult time deciding to change my last name, as I came to consider it a strength. It was only in writing this book and reflecting on my identity that I've been able to acknowledge that my identity is (and can be) ever-changing.

Depending on what facet of identity you want to examine—gender, race, sexual orientation, living with a disability—you may be on a spectrum of privileged to marginalized, based on your background with several factors being outside of your control. If you are privileged, you may be completely unaware of the differences in opportunities that exist. If you identify as marginalized, you may be acutely aware of these differences. For someone with mixed heritage who appears Caucasian, I often go about my days completely unaware of any discrimination, but I am conscious anytime an application asks if I "identify as anything other than Caucasian." I will then find myself weighing the pros and cons of checking yes to other, and typing in "Armenian."

Wherever you fall on the spectrum, this section is for you because awareness of your identity is important.

We know that identifying as a member of a marginalized group can come with disadvantages in many facets of life. Nurses value equity and inclusiveness. Alas, certain biases can be unconscious and entrenched—which may feel beyond your control. I want to focus on what is *in your control*; to make your unique identity *a strength*.

The goal is to identify areas that you can flip from negative to positive, or double down on if they are already positive. I want you to feel confident in your skin and identity. Doing this exercise will help you be a step ahead in your interactions with employers, managers, patients, or other clients. Consider it part of your self-marketing plan.

For example, having an accent can be seen as either a strength or a weakness. Walking into a job interview you can either:

1. Not call attention to your accent;
2. Give short answers for fewer opportunities for your accent to be heard; or,
3. Start the conversation by acknowledging your accent, and highlighting how your knowledge of a second language can benefit an employer by being able to better serve patients who would otherwise have difficulty accessing nursing services.

Option one leaves it to the other party to determine whether your accent is a strength or weakness. Option two will likely result in selling yourself short, as you may come off as timid in a nursing position that requires you to interact with people daily. Meanwhile, option three cuts any tension, invites the other party to get to know you and your background, and presents your unique accent as a strength. By planning ahead and owning this unique quality, you get to be in control of the narrative.

If you can't find an employer who appreciates your unique identity, consider building a business of your own. You will have no one to answer to but yourself and, you will 100% find clients who appreciate your perspective, your take on a problem, your personality, and the solutions that only *you* can provide based on your unique life experiences. If you need financial or educational support while starting your business there are an abundant number of supports for individuals who identify as part of a marginalized groups.

You have the power to harness your unique strengths to do great things in the world of nursing. Don't hold yourself back any more than the world conspires to, instead keep your strengths at the forefront of your mind as you move forward in your nursing career.

EXERCISE: Your Unique Strengths

Write a list of qualities that you love about yourself, that you may hold back in social or professional settings for fear of judgment. Next, think about examples of your identity helping you, as well as holding you back. If this task is emotional, consider enlisting professional help for a deeper dive.

NURSING WISELY: STORIES FROM SUCCESSFUL NURSES

"In learning from the stories of others, we unlock a treasure trove of wisdom, experiences, and perspectives that can shape our own journey."

—Unknown

Four nurses. Four different paths of women having a successful career on their own terms.

Claudia Mariano, Former Nurse Practitioner

Claudia Mariano is a retired Nurse Practitioner with over three decades of experience. Her focus was primary care with clients across the lifespan with special interest in chronic disease management, diabetes, and smoking cessation. In addition to clinical experience, she worked to ensure self-regulation and accountability of Nurse Practitioners, and has extensive experience working with healthcare organizations and external stakeholders such as government and policy makers. She is the author/editor of, *No One Left Behind: How Nurse Practitioners Are Changing Canada's Health Care System*.

Q: Do you consider yourself to have had a successful nursing career?

I am fortunate to have had a varied career with many opportunities and feel overall that my career path has been very successful.

Q: Do you feel your nursing career was worthwhile? In what way(s)?

While nursing as a career has its challenges, my career offered me many options in a variety of roles that I was able to pivot as my life circumstances changed. For example, as a new mother and student, I was able to work part-time and take contract positions that supported my schedule yet still allowed time for my growing family and educational pursuits. Later on, I was able to work full-time in supportive environments that allowed me to further develop my skills and obtain other certifications (as a diabetes educator and also in smoking cessation).

Q: Did your nursing career pursuits interest you and keep your attention? If yes, how did you maintain this? If not, how did you persevere?

I believe this is one of the most critical aspects of nursing as a career. The options are only limited by one's own vision and determination. I was able to participate, not only as an expert clinician with patients, but I also pursued opportunities to present at conferences and participate in professional advocacy through my professional association, NPAO, as well as other organizations. I believe nurses bring a critical perspective to health policy tables that is often lacking. Taking advantage of opportunities for broader stakeholder engagement provided constant new opportunities to keep me engaged and learning.

Q: Do you feel your nursing career is something you can see yourself pursuing beyond traditional retirement?

While I consider myself recently retired, I am fortunate to remain closely connected to the NP community. I am excited to see that younger NPs (and others who are more experienced) have an entrepreneurial flair and social media savvy that makes them more able to pivot to non-traditional nursing roles as business owners and entrepreneurs. While there is division in our profession when it comes to patients paying for nursing services, this new growth area illustrates how quickly nurses are able to identify gaps and pivot to fill them in. This challenge to the status quo will generate conversation about the state of our health care system and what we, as a profession and society, want to support.

Q: Did your nursing career have boundaries or limiting beliefs? If so, how did you overcome them?

Personally, I don't feel I had any limiting beliefs for my career, as I didn't see it as one straight line but as a tree firmly rooted in nursing with many branches that I could pick from as my life circumstances changed. This provided me with a broad perspective and experience which I feel was valued by employers and stakeholders.

Q: What would you change about your career, if anything?

My nursing career allowed me to put my family and personal growth first, which kept me energized and excited about patient care.

Dr. Sonja Mitrevska Schwartzbach, CRNA

Dr. Sonja Mitrevska Schwartzbach is a Certified Registered Nurse Anesthetist (CRNA) and Advanced Practice Nurse with over a decade of nursing experience. With a background in English Literature before becoming a nurse, Dr. Schwartzbach fulfilled a goal by her thirtieth birthday of becoming a published author. Her first book, *Oh Sh*t, I Almost Killed You! A Little Book of Big Things Nursing School Forgot to Teach You* has sold over 150,000 copies. She has written on behalf of numerous nursing and lifestyle outlets including "The Huffington Post." Her second book, *Coffee with My Dead Mother: Lessons on Loss, Hope, and Navigating a New Normal* was published March 2022, followed by *You Won't Feel a Thing: The Drama, Tragedy, Camp; Comedy of Healthcare*" in September 2022. You can follow her on Instagram at @nursesonja.

Q: Do you consider yourself to have had a successful nursing career?

Yes and no. The profession of nursing requires strict boundaries. As a natural empath, I often found myself feeling guilted into extra shifts, staying late, and skipping breaks. If the provider I am today could give any advice to "new nurse" me, it would be to find a way to distinguish your role in healthcare from your identity. I believe I have evolved into a skilled and capable anesthesia provider, and that I will always maintain the core tenets of compassion in my care…but at times, that came with a price.

Q: Do you feel your nursing career is/was worthwhile?

I am forever grateful for my decision to leave my corporate career and become a nurse, even more so now as a doctoral prepared certified registered nurse anesthetist (CRNA). The value of the nursing profession stems in its depth and breadth. A career in nursing is highly transferrable, and whether you choose to practice within an acute care setting or never set foot inside of a hospital, the core tenets of critical thinking, analysis, reading, writing, and interdisciplinary interaction will carry you into any sector of the nursing field.

Q: Did your nursing career keep your attention?

The truth is, I am easily bored and intensely curious. The progression from being a seasoned intensive care unit nurse into anesthesia felt like a natural next step for me, and in many ways that is because of my own quest for knowledge and advancement. One of my favorite parts (and one of the greatest challenges) about anesthesia is that no two patients or cases are alike. It is an intensely humbling field, and the growth and expansion of technology and intervention keeps my attention every day.

Q: Do you feel your nursing career is something you can see yourself pursuing beyond traditional retirement?

I don't intend to do anything "traditionally." Retirement included.

Q: Is/was your career empowered? Is/was lifelong learning a key component of your career empowerment strategy?

Yes and no. In truth, I felt limited in my career as a bedside nurse due to systemic issues that couldn't be challenged or readily changed. It was not until I branched out of my role as a nurse and became a published author that I stepped into my power...because if I didn't take ownership for my voice, who would? I believe that education is crucial but even the most adept learner will hit systems-based roadblocks. Therefore, self-awareness is crucial in determining how you choose to frame your professional role. What matters more to you: stability or taking risks? Feeling comfortable or the unknown? Being a team member or being your own boss?

Q: Does/did your nursing career have boundaries? If so, how did you overcome them?

Every single member of the nursing profession faces boundaries, and these limitations are placed by the financial chokeholds placed upon providers by institutions. The moment that healthcare became a for-profit landscape, nursing became the group to suffer, to bear the brunt of the burden, to endure staffing cuts, budgetary changes, and algorithmic care. In truth, I fought until I could no longer do so and preserve my desire to remain in healthcare. My decision to walk away from bedside was not without my own (fruitless) battles with the powers at be.

Q: Does/did your nursing career come from a place of authenticity? What might you change about your career, if anything?

My segue into nursing came from a passion to care for others the way my family members had been cared for. Would I do it again? No. Likely not. At least, not given the current landscape of healthcare and mistreatment of nurses as a whole. Having witnessed the manipulation of natural empaths in order to turn a profit, I would not enter the profession again...or at least, not without a plan to leave the bedside within a reasonable time frame. I love what I do and am grateful for a rewarding career as a nurse anesthetist, but I loved being an ICU nurse. I was great at it. My role inspired me, but it also burned me out. It stole pieces of myself that can never be returned. If I could do it all again, I would set firm boundaries from the very start, in order to preserve my peace and protect my wellness. You are not your job. Do not accept the notion that the building will crumble without you. It will not. They will figure it out, as they always do. Put yourself first, and you will ultimately become a better provider for it.

Melane Mullings

Melane Mullings is a successful entrepreneur, cancer survivor, former registered nurse, founder of Aere Management Consulting, an award-winning author, and TEDx speaker. Melane's cancer journey provided her a deep understanding of the foundations of success which she extrapolated to her first entrepreneurial venture in the healthcare recruiting space. Thirteen years after establishing her nursing recruitment firm, Melane sold her business, and is now sharing her unconventional, yet proven strategies to success in her #1 bestselling book: *Lemonade! Squeeze Your Challenging Life Experiences into a Successful Business*, and through her business management consulting practice, *Aere Management Consulting*. Her consultancy grants her the opportunity to help struggling business owners transition to a state of sustained profitability, build a solid foundation for growth, and learn strategies to enjoy an improved quality of life as a business owner. Prior to starting her business ventures, Melane graduated with honors from Queen's University in Canada with a Bachelor of Nursing Science degree, and worked as a Registered Nurse in both the United States and Canada. Melane is an active volunteer, philanthropist, Board member of the Canadian organization, *Immigrant Women in Business*, and a mentor with *Futurpreneur Canada*. Her motto:

"go boldly, dare greatly, love passionately, live intentionally" fully encapsulates her approach to life.

Q: Do you consider yourself to have had a successful nursing career?

Yes, I do. I stopped renewing my license a few years back but, in my mind, I'll always be a nurse.

Q: Do you feel your nursing career was worthwhile? In what way(s)?

It helped me launch my nursing recruitment firm and gave me perspective on the Canadian health system and the needs and desires of nurses. I wouldn't have been able to operate my nursing staffing business effectively without that knowledge. Nursing didn't make me. Surviving leukemia informed how I developed. As a young person, I thought like a nurse—with compassion and accountability. Nursing allowed me to explore more of who I was.

Q: Did your nursing career pursuits interest you and keep your attention?

No, nursing was a stage on my purpose journey. There was a point I suffered burnout, I wasn't happy and my work wasn't fulfilling. I was not operating to the full scope of my purpose.

Q: Do you consider your career to be empowered?

Lifelong learning and the concept of "Kaizen," a Japanese word meaning continuous improvement have been central themes in my career. Whether I learned this in nursing I cannot say. Did a nursing career empower me? Yes. As a graduate from Queen's University, you are imbued with the idea of continuous improvement. With CARNA licensure you are encouraged to continue your learning. I can't say that came from nursing education initially, but it became part of my life and now, I teach my clients about the importance of continuous improvement to grow their businesses. We should all be learning on a continuum.

Q: Did your nursing career have boundaries or limiting beliefs? If so, how did you overcome them?

I wouldn't blame nursing culture as having boundaries, but did experience limiting perspectives among the seasoned nurses who I was exposed to early in my career. While at Queen's I was taught about the many career opportunities available to me as a nurse. I absolutely *did not* see the career as constraining. There were no limiting beliefs in my education. Unfortunately, some of the people I worked with early in my career *were* infected with limiting beliefs, but I overcame that by staying true to my purpose and leaning on my Christian faith. Now, as a consultant, I help people understand their "why." I help them answer the questions: Why am I here? What are my skills and passions, and how can I use them (as well as other challenging life experiences) to live an abundant, fulfilling, impactful life? Answering those questions helped me unlock my purpose, and persevere toward creating a life of meaning and impact for myself.

Q: Did your nursing career come from a place of authenticity and meet your needs first? If not, what might you change about your career?

My career was an extension of who I was. From the time I survived Leukemia, I became a nurse in my mind. Did it meet my needs? Initially, it did. I had a successful career as a per diem and travel nurse, making six figures in my 20s, but it did not fulfill my purpose. The position of floor nurse also didn't serve my greater purpose but it met my financial needs and was a step on my journey. I wouldn't change anything in my career except that I would've liked to spend more time working as an ER nurse. I stayed long enough to understand the healthcare system and the conditions that nurses face. It fostered my compassion to create job opportunities for nurses, and to recruit from that perspective. (What I would change about the healthcare system is an entirely different question!) It comes down to finding an area that you love. Move around. Don't sit in a position where you are burnt out.

There are many options, and the system needs nurses to stay— which I supported through the operation of my recruitment firm. Bringing nurses to the healthcare system was a fulfilling step along the road of my purpose journey. My takeaway is this: take the time to find what you love. If it is nursing, explore the various opportunities available to you as a nurse; they are so vast! Commit to working in the capacity that feeds your passion and draws from your inherent skills. There is where you'll have the greatest impact, find enjoyment in your work, and experience fulfillment in your role.

Stacey Roles, RN MScN PhD Psychotherapist

Stacey Roles (she/her) is an Academy of Cognitive Therapy (ACT) Certified Trainer Consultant and Certified Cognitive Therapist and is also credentialed with the Canadian Association of Cognitive and Behavioural Therapies (CACBT). Stacey has advanced training and supervision in prolonged exposure therapy and compassion focused therapy. Stacey is competent in treating clients across the lifespan from early childhood to older adults. She is an Adjunct Professor at Laurentian University with the School of Nursing and was associate CBT lead for the advanced CBT lectures in the psychiatry residency program at the Northern Ontario School of Medicine University where she currently holds the rank of Assistant Professor. Stacey has extensive experience working with First Nations populations throughout Ontario specifically in the remote and rural Northern Ontario.

Stacey Roles, RN PhD specializes in providing consulting services to those who work with complex mental health presentations, in both large and small organizations. Stacey has extensive experience consulting with mental health clinicians and supportive staff in Indigenous communities and offers an assortment of other specialized or advanced learning and consulting needs. Stacey leads the CBT Training Centre of the North and Roles & Associates Psychotherapy Services Inc.

Q: Do you consider yourself to have or to have had a successful nursing career?

Yes, very much so. I began nursing when I graduated from a three-year college RN program in 2003 at Cambrian college in Sudbury, ON and very shortly after that started in psychiatry in a mental health inpatient unit in London Ontario. From then I spent the majority of my career working inpatient and outpatient mental health, in pharmacy departments, teaching at med schools and in nursing programs and training groups in psychotherapy, such as cognitive behavioural therapy and compassion-focused therapy. From there, I built my own practice with currently about 15 associates and have a successful psychotherapy and workshop training company.

Q: Do you feel your nursing career is/was worthwhile?

Yes. There's been a lot of challenges, particularly when insurance companies, governments and the public devalue the role of nursing. This has been a particular struggle for nurse psychotherapists, and independent practice nurses but I think we've come a long way. Having a nursing background and knowing the medical component and how health systems work has been extremely worthwhile to me. I have been a clinical educator and clinical nurse specialist in different systems which helped me learn how to write policies and understand healthcare, medicine, pharmacology and nursing interventions. Furthermore, the nurse client relationship and rapport building in psychotherapy or any client interaction is something that very few professions would have such comprehensive learning opportunities, so I definitely feel that my nursing career was worthwhile.

Q: Do/did your nursing career pursuits interest you and keep your attention?

Nursing is one of those professions that I believe gets devalued because outsiders view of nursing is often so broad. This perspective tends to give the impression that "a nurse is a nurse is a nurse," and that nurses don't specialize. The view of a nurse as a generalist allows nurses to dive into any area or specialty within the profession. The problem, as I see it, is once you get there it's difficult for people to see us as experts in our niche. Nursing stayed interesting because I was able to pursue different avenues, particularly diving in as a specialist in psychotherapies, and persevering through the changes in the recognition that needed to happen as an entrepreneur, and as an RN PhD psychotherapist. Luckily, because of a collective of like-minded nurses who had the same pursuit of excellence in nursing as I have, I've been supported to advance the nursing profession in psychotherapy.

Q: Do you feel your nursing career is something you can see yourself pursuing beyond traditional retirement?

Yes, because I've already left traditional nursing, having worked within hospital systems for almost 20 years of my career. Being the owner and director of my own private practice, has changed what normal retirement looks like. Having the flexibility to make my own hours and schedule my own vacation time, not having to ask (or beg) for time off has been extremely freeing. I love what I do. I love consulting, supervising and teaching people psychotherapy and helping therapists to become better at what they do. I love doing intensive psychotherapy sessions for clients and helping people recover from what they're struggling with. For these reasons I could definitely see myself doing this beyond the traditional idea of "putting your years in" before retirement.

Q: Is/was your career empowered? Is/was lifelong learning a key component of your career empowerment strategy?

My career is very empowered thanks to the many like-minded nurses and other mental health professionals that I've met along the way. One area where I've engaged in lifelong learning has been in the pursuit of my graduate degrees. I completed my PhD in 2021. Beyond that, I've studied different psychotherapies, and am currently co-editing and writing a book on nursing and psychotherapy. It has felt empowering to help other nurses to follow similar career paths.

Q: Did your nursing career have limiting beliefs? If so, how did you overcome them?

My nursing career had *a lot* of limiting beliefs. At first, the idea that I'd have to work as a nurse on a floor for my entire career, was difficult and it impacted my interest in wanting to stay in the profession. The shift work, and lack of autonomy that I experienced made it difficult to picture myself staying there until retirement. I was hopeful that I would find my passion, and I was lucky that I found it early in my career and have been able to continue to develop it. The work I do now enables me to interact with clinicians working with clients on inpatient units, outpatient departments and private practices with all sorts of presentations, diagnoses and symptoms. In this way I'm really getting to use all the years of my almost twenty years of nursing experience. I am very fortunate that some limiting beliefs and boundaries have been lifted, but a lot of them were trails that my colleagues and myself had to blaze. We're hoping that we've made it a little bit easier for nurses—especially nurse psychotherapists.

Q: Does/did your nursing career come from a place of authenticity and meet your needs?

Going into nursing came naturally for me as there are many nurses in my family. I always considered myself a compassionate person and enjoyed helping others. The way in which I helped others needed to be from a place of my own autonomy, rather than feeling as though I was being assigned tasks based on a system around me. One part that I struggled with from the beginning wasn't so much the shift work itself, but rather the lack of ability to take time off for family events. Having to ask (or in many cases plead with) management or other nurses to cover work shifts was very off putting. That restriction on work/life balance was a big motivator to get out of that type of structured system, and into a place where I had weekends off. Working within a hospital, but dayshift Monday to Friday, was better but the same feelings of frustration would arise when I would be declined vacation time or questioned for taking an allotted sick day. Some organizations don't function this way, and many are struggling with a nursing shortage, but in the positions, I was working in —this was the reality. I wish I'd known that it was okay to leave a job that wasn't well-suited for me because of work/life balance reasons. At the same time, I wouldn't change any of it because it led me to this place in my career where I am fulfilled.

EPILOGUE

This was the book I was meant to write and this was the book *you* were meant to read! But, what next? As the saying goes, "What's for you, won't go past you."

The future may be unclear, but know that you are smart, capable and worthy of a career that is fulfilling and lucrative. No matter what decade of life or stage of career you're in, it is time for you to write your next chapter. You have a vision for your nursing career and new tools at your disposal. Now, I challenge you to take inspired action.

Worthwhile. You've discovered what makes your nursing career worthwhile! You've built career goals inspired by your values and vision!

Interesting. Keep your career interesting! Adopt a curious mindset and seize aligned opportunities, challenges, and learning opportunities.

Sustainable. Build a career that is sustainable! Get to work creating a network of supportive colleagues, organizations, and even government officials. Grow your support system deep and wide like the roots of trees. Maintain momentum and build a career that creates a legacy beyond yourself. Join the *Nursing WISELY* community or build a support circle of your own.

Empowered. Follow the roadmap to empowerment! You are no ordinary nurse—you are armed with the knowledge to influence the lives of many people who need your expertise. Trust your gut and put your dreams ahead of your fears.

Limitless. You've examined your limiting beliefs! You know there is no limit on your capacity for improvement.

You. Put yourself first! Make a promise to yourself that you will embrace your unique strengths, honour your authentic self, prioritize your own well-being, and prioritize your personal growth and fulfillment.

Not sure what to do next? Here is your first step: Rate yourself *again* on the Nursing WISELY career success scale. Then, *take action* in your biggest area of opportunity. Revisit relevant chapters in this book as needed, or reread it in its entirety. Who knows what you may have missed the first time around!

Make the next twelve months count.

Thank you!

Your dedication to the nursing profession has been the inspiration behind this book. I hope you've found comfort in these pages, as well as understanding and a reflection of your own experiences. Now, I kindly ask you to share this journey with your fellow nurses.

Recommend *Nursing WISELY* to your colleagues and friends. Together, let's create a ripple effect, sparking conversations and strengthening our nursing community. Your support in spreading the word *will* make an impact.

Thank you for embarking on this transformative journey with me. Harness the wisdom you've gained in reading this book to enhance your life and the lives of all nurses. Illuminate the profound power of nursing to the world!

BONUS: ORGANIZATIONAL RECRUITMENT AND RETENTION WITH *NURSING WISELY*

HEALTHCARE ORGANIZATIONS AND NURSE LEADERS have one thing in common: you need nurses. Recruiting, training, and retaining nurses is an expensive process. What is even more expensive is nurse turnover. So, how do you prevent turnover? Use Nursing *WISELY*.

If you're not a nurse leader (yet), gift a copy to a nurse leader who you think could benefit from the principles of Nursing WISELY and move the needle for your nursing colleagues.

Each of the six areas of the Nursing WISELY paradigm corresponds to an area that you can influence and address to improve your nursing staff satisfaction and retention. Explore each module with your nursing staff to determine areas for opportunity. Use this tool to help you better understand how to support your staff, spot red flags, and address issues before you lose valuable staff members.

Leaders are responsible for motivating staff toward a common goal. Each module of Nursing WISELY can be influenced - positively and negatively. Explore how leadership can influence a move toward the impact your organization seeks to achieve.

EXERCISE: Rate Your Organization

Rate your organization on a scale of 1 to 10, where 1 is not at all and 10 is absolutely.

Periodically return to this rating scale to assess areas of strength and opportunity in your organization.

My organizational goals create an environment where a nursing career can feel worthwhile and allow nursing staff to be guided toward nursing career opportunities that are meaningful, valuable and aligned with personal values.

①—②—③—④—⑤—⑥—⑦—⑧—⑨—⑩

My organization provides career opportunities that keep nursing staff engaged.

①—②—③—④—⑤—⑥—⑦—⑧—⑨—⑩

My organization provides nursing career opportunities that nursing staff can see themselves pursuing into retirement and beyond.

①—②—③—④—⑤—⑥—⑦—⑧—⑨—⑩

My organization enables career development and growth through access to resources, mentorship programs, training opportunities and autonomy to practice to full scope.

①—②—③—④—⑤—⑥—⑦—⑧—⑨—⑩

My organization encourages nurses to pursue limitless career aspirations by fostering a supportive environment.

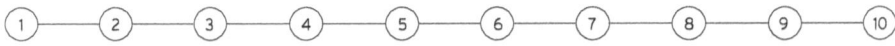

My organization encourages nursing staff to practice from a place of authenticity, meeting their needs first.

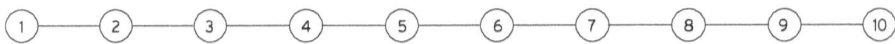

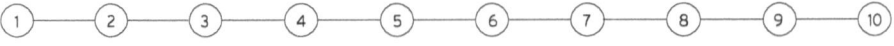

For anything you rated less than 10, what is one thing you can do to bring your organization closer to a 10?

SELECTED BIBLIOGRAPHY / WORKS CITED

Hershfield, H. E., Goldstein, D. G., Sharpe, W. F., Fox, J., Yeykelis, L., Carstensen, L. L., & Bailenson, J. N. (2011). Increasing Saving Behavior Through Age-Progressed Renderings of the Future Self. *Journal of Marketing Research*, 48(SPL), S23–S37. https://doi.org/10.1509/jmkr.48.SPL.S23

Bravata, D. M., Watts, S. A., Keefer, A. L., Madhusudhan, D. K., Taylor, K. T., Clark, D. M., Nelson, R. S., Cokley, K. O., & Hagg, H. K. (2020). Prevalence, Predictors, and Treatment of Impostor Syndrome: a Systematic Review. *Journal of general internal medicine*, 35(4), 1252–1275. https://doi.org/10.1007/s11606-019-05364-1

Clance, P. R., & Imes, S. A. (1978). The imposter phenomenon in high achieving women: Dynamics and therapeutic intervention. *Psychotherapy: Theory, Research & Practice*, 15(3), 241–247. https://doi.org/10.1037/h0086006

Cleary, M., Sayers, J., Lopez, V. & Hungerford, C. (2016). Boredom in the Workplace: Reasons, Impact, and Solutions, *Issues in Mental Health Nursing*, 37:2, 83-89, DOI: 10.3109/01612840.2015.1084554

McMillan, D. & Fallis, W. (2011). Benefits of napping on night shifts. *Nursing Times* [online]; 107: 44, 12-13.

Holiday, Ryan. (2014). *The Obstacle Is the Way: The Timeless Art of Turning Trials Into Triumph*. Portfolio.

Iconomopoulos, Fotini. (2021). *Say Less, Get More: Unconventional Negotiation Techniques to Get What You Want*. Collins.

Lorsch, J. W., & Morse, J. J. (1985). Career paths and career success in the early career stages of male and female MBAs. *Journal of Organizational Behavior*, 6(4), 289-306.

Mariano, C. (2015). *No One Left behind: How Nurse Practitioners Are Changing the Canadian Health Care System*. Friesen Press, Inc.

Maslow, A. H. (1954). *Motivation and personality*. New York: Harper and Row.

Mullings, Melane. (2022). *Lemonade!: Squeeze Your Challenging Life Experiences into a Successful Business*. Aere Management Consulting.

Schwartzbach, S. (2017). *Oh Sh*t, I Almost Killed You! A Little Book of Big Things Nursing School Forgot to Teach You*. Sonja M. Schwartzbach.

Sinek, S. (2011). *Start with WHY: How great leaders inspire everyone to take action*. Penguin Books.

Stampfer, M. J., & Schernhammer, E. S. (2016). Association Between Rotating Night Shift Work and Risk of Coronary Heart Disease Among Women. *JAMA*, 315(16), 1726–1734. https://doi.org/10.1001/jama.2016.4454

Sundström, A., Rönnlund, M., & Josefsson, M. (2020). A nationwide Swedish study of age at retirement and dementia risk. *International Journal of Geriatric Psychiatry*, 35(10), 1243-1249.

Syamlal, G., Doney, B., Hendricks, S., & Mazurek, J.M. (2021). Chronic obstructive pulmonary disease and U.S. workers: prevalence, trends, and attributable cases associated with work. *Am J Prev Med*, 61(3):e127-e137. https://doi:10.1016/j.amepre.2021.04.011

Van Manen, M. (2014). *Phenomenology of Practice*. Walnut Creek, CA: Left Coast Press, Inc.

Vetter, C., Devore, E. E., Wegrzyn, L. R., Massa, J., Speizer, F. E., Kawachi, I., Rosner, B., & Walker, L.E. (1984). *The Battered Woman Syndrome*. New York, Springer Publishing Company.

Villeneuve, M. (2017). *Public Policy and Canadian Nursing: Lessons from the Field*. Canadian Scholars.

Zwicky, A. M. (2006). Why are we so illuded? Retrieved January 28, 2023 from http://www-csli.stanford.edu/~ zwicky/LSA07illude.abst.pdf.

Are you feeling overwhelmed?

Charged and excited?

Send me your comments, reactions, personal stories,
or good advice for others!

Follow me at **http://www.maryghazarian.com/**
for more support and tips.

Pay it forward. Write a review on Amazon
and gift a copy of this book!

ABOUT THE AUTHOR

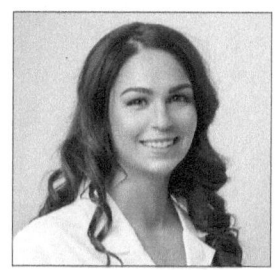

Mary Ghazarian, MN, NP-PHC, is a dynamic nurse leader with a passion for inspiring positive change, advancing the nursing profession, and improving patient outcomes through the sharing of knowledge and innovation.

Mary holds a Baccalaureate degree from Queen's University in Kingston, Ontario, and a Master's degree in Nursing with a Primary Health Care Nurse Practitioner certification from Ryerson University (now named Toronto Metropolitan University).

Through her passion for nurse career coaching, Mary utilizes her extensive expertise to empower nurses in achieving their professional goals and creating fulfilling careers. Alongside her clinical practice, she has made significant contributions as an accomplished author, engaging speaker, and dedicated educator—inspiring positive change and driving growth within the nursing profession.

Mary's commitment to guiding nurses to excel and thrive has established her as a trusted mentor and advocate for professional success.

www.ingramcontent.com/pod-product-compliance
Lightning Source LLC
Chambersburg PA
CBHW031104080526
44587CB00011B/816